SPINAL NARCOTICS

CURRENT MANAGEMENT OF PAIN

P. PRITHVI RAJ, SERIES EDITOR

The series, *Current Management of Pain*, is intended by the series editor and the publishers to provide up-to-date information on advances in the clinical management of acute and chronic pain and related research as quickly as possible. Both the series editor and the publishers felt that, although comprehensive texts are now available, they do not always cover the rapid advances in this field. Another format was needed to publish advances in basic sciences and clinical modalities and to bring them rapidly to the practitioners in the community. A questionnaire was sent to selected clinicians and, based on their responses, topics were chosen by the series editor. Editors of each volume were chosen for their expertise in the field and their ability to encourage other active pain specialists to contribute their knowledge:

Ghia, J.N., ed.: The Multidisciplinary Pain Center: Organization and Personnel Functions for Pain Management, 1988. ISBN 0-89838-359-5.

Lynch, N.T., Vasudevan, S.V., eds.: Persistent Pain: Psychosocial Assessment and Intervention, 1988. ISBN 0-89838-363-3.

Abram, S.E., ed.: Cancer Pain, 1988. ISBN 0-89838-389-7.

Racz, G.B., ed.: Techniques of Neurolysis, 1989. ISBN 0-89838-397-8.

Stanton-Hicks, M., ed.: Pain and the Sympathetic Nervous System, 1989. ISBN 0-7923-0304-0

Rawal, N., Coombs, D.W., eds.: Spinal Narcotics, 1990. ISBN 0-7923-0374-1.

SPINAL NARCOTICS

Edited by
NARINDER RAWAL AND DENNIS W. COOMBS

KLUWER ACADEMIC PUBLISHERS
BOSTON DORDRECHT LONDON

Distributors
for North America: Kluwer Academic Publishers, 101 Philip Drive, Assinippi Park, Norwell, Massachusetts 02061 USA

for all other countries:, Kluwer Academic Publishers Group, Distribution Centre, Post Office Box 322, 3300 AH Dordrecht, The Netherlands

Library of Congress Cataloging-in-Publication Data
Spinal Narcotics / edited by Narinder Rawal, Dennis W. Coombs.
p. cm. — (Current management of pain ; 6)
Includes index.
ISBN 0-7923-0374-1
1. Spinal anesthesia. 2. Endorphins — Receptors. 3. Narcotics.
I. Rawal, Narinder. II. Coombs, Dennis W. III. Series.
[DNLM: 1. Anesthesia, Spinal. 2. Narcotics — pharmacology.
3. Narcotics — therapeutic use. 4. Pain — drug therapy.
5. Receptors, Endorphin. WO 305 S757]
RD85.S7S63 1989
617.9'64 — dc20
DNLM/DLC
for Library of Congress 89-15480
CIP

PRINTED IN THE UNITED STATES OF AMERICA.

CONTENTS

CONTENTS

Contributing authors vii

Series editor foreword ix

Preface xi

1. Opioid receptors: Types, distribution, and pharmacological profiles 1
   THOMAS HEDNER, GUNNAR NORDBERG
2. Systemic and local distribution of opioids after spinal administration: Implications for their clinical use 33
   LARS L. GUSTAFSSON
3. Indications for the use of intraspinal opioids 43
   NARINDER RAWAL
4. Perioperative stress reduction with intraspinal opioids 63
   MARK YEAGER
5. Adverse effects of spinal opioids in acute pain and their management 77
   NARINDER RAWAL
6. The role of intraspinal opioids in obstetrics 89
   SAMUEL C. HUGHES
7. Delivery systems for chronic spinal analgesia 115
   DENNIS W. COOMBS
8. Spinal opioid analgesia: Present status and future developments 129
   PERRY G. FINE, THEODORE H. STANLEY

Index 145

CONTRIBUTING AUTHORS

Dennis W. Coombs, M.D., Editor
Assistant Professor of Anesthesiology
Dartmouth Medical School
Dartmouth-Hitchcock Medical Center
Hanover, NH 03756, U.S.A.

Perry G. Fine, M.D.
Assistant Professor
Department of Anesthesiology
University of Utah Medical Center
Salt Lake City, UT 84132, U.S.A.

Lars L. Gustafsson, M.D., Ph.D.
Senior Clinical Associate
Department of Clinical Pharmacology
Huddinge University Hospital
Karolinska Institute
Stockholm, Sweden

Thomas Hedner, M.D., Ph.D.
Associate Professor
Department of Clinical Pharmacology
Sahlgrenska University Hospital
Gothenburg, Sweden

Samuel C. Hughes, M.D.
Assistant Clinical Professor
Department of Anesthesia
San Francisco General Hospital
San Francisco, CA 94143-0410, U.S.A.

Gunnar Nordberg, M.D., Ph.D.
Senior Consultant Anesthetist
Department of Anesthesiology
Sahlgrenska University Hospital
Gothenburg, Sweden

Narinder Rawal, M.D., Ph.D., Editor
Senior Consultant Anesthetist
Department of Anesthesiology and Intensive Care
Orebro Medical Center Hospital
Orebro, Sweden
and
Visiting Professor
Department of Anesthesiology
University of Texas Medical School at Houston
Houston, TX 77030, U.S.A.

Theodore H. Stanley, M.D.
Professor of Anesthesiology
Department of Anesthesiology
School of Medicine
University at Utah Medical Center
Salt Lake City, UT 84132, U.S.A.

Mark Yeager, M.D.
Assistant Professor
Department of Anesthesiology
Dartmouth Medical School
Dartmouth-Hitchcock Medical Center
Hanover, NH 03756, U.S.A.

SERIES EDITOR FOREWORD

One of the most exciting developments in medicine in this century has been the discovery of opioid receptors and their pharmacology. The breadth of knowledge derived from such discovery has truly changed the practice of medicine today. The acceptance by the clinicians of the research data obtained by the basic scientist on spinal opioids is truly amazing. The clinical sequelae of the discovery of opioid receptors has been the development of the technique of intraspinal administration of opioids. In the last decade much has been written about indications, effects, and side effects of intraspinal opioids. The technique has become commonplace for cancer and postoperative pain. However, no standards of care and management of patients with spinally administered opioids have been developed. We need these standards to be developed and universally followed.

The monograph was conceived to update clinicians on the applied pharmacology of spinal opioids. We were fortunate to have Drs. N. Rawal and D. Coombs agree to edit this monograph. They have been able to assemble world-renowned experts as contributing authors. It is our hope that the contents of this book will be stimulating, informative, and useful to the reader.

PREFACE

Much has been written about the subject of spinal opioid analgesia, including several notable reviews. We were stimulated to assemble this particular volume in this important series on pain management initiated by Dr. Raj for a number of reasons. Our first intention was simply to update the anesthesiologists working in pain management. However, this series clearly is intended for other specialists working in the same area. Our hope is that the balance of basic and clinical science is such that the clinician/scientist other than the anesthesiologist may also benefit from the collected subjects.

We have attempted to cover certain "new" areas, such as spinal opioid infusions and modulation of surgical and postoperative stress responses, and to update both basic and clinical aspects of spinal opioid analgesia. The chapter by Fine and Stanley reflects an interesting perspective on the general direction that we may be taking in the 1990s.

Stylistic differences and some overlap are inevitable in a multi-authored monograph of this nature, and for this we apologize. Throughout this volume, the term *opioid* is used to denote both endogenous and exogenous agents and agonists exerting effects upon opioid (opiate) receptors regardless of their site or action. The term *intraspinal* has been employed as a generic equivalent to both epidural and intrathecal. Similarly, *epidural* has been utilized throughout for extradural or peridural and intrathecal; *subarachnoid* and *spinal* are favored over intradural.

We gratefully acknowledge the efforts of the individual authors for their timely contributions, the editorial assistance of Marilyn Schwiers, our secretaries, Betty Cunha and Katherine Dow, and finally, our series editor, P. Raj, for his many thoughtful suggestions and avuncular attitude.

SPINAL NARCOTICS

1. OPIOID RECEPTORS: TYPES, DISTRIBUTION, AND PHARMACOLOGICAL PROFILES

THOMAS HEDNER AND GUNNAR NORDBERG

Although the use of opium can be traced back to the ancient Sumerians [1] and the receptor theory of drug actions was proposed at the turn of the century [2], the actual postulation and demonstration of distinct receptor binding sites for morphine and other opiates was first made in 1973 through the work of Pert and Snyder [3], Simon et al. [4], and Terenius [5]. Several prior decades of studies of opiate pharmacology had outlined but not formulated the idea of specific binding sites. Such studies included, e.g., demonstration of rigid structural requirements for drug action, stereospecificity, and dose-dependent actions, as well as the existence of specific antagonists [6].

An early first breakthrough for the modern concept of opiate analgesia originated with two Chineses scientists, Tsou and Jang [7]. In 1964, they showed that minute amounts of morphine produced analgesia when injected into a discrete area of the rabbit brain, the periventricular gray. These findings were later confirmed and extended in several laboratories around the world [8–11], and a specific spinal site of opiate action was also outlined [10–12]. Such brain areas, intimately involved in opiate analgesic action, were subsequently demonstrated to possess specific and high-affinity opiate binding sites [3–5, 13–15]. The establishment of specific receptor sites upon which opiates acted stimulated the speculation and search for endogenous structures that might act as ligands on the specific receptor sites. Such evidence was obtained by Terenius and Wahlström [16]. Nearly simultaneously, the structures of the enkephalins were presented by Hughes et al. [17], β-endorphin by Bradbury et al. [18] and Li and Chung [19], and, somewhat later, the dynorphin structure by Goldstein et al. [20]. Since then, the intense research efforts in this area have resulted in the discovery of multiple peripheral and central endogenous opioid peptides, as well as a multiplicity of receptors. This expansion revealed not only the complexity of the central and peripheral opioid systems but also created an abundance of nomenclature [21, 22]. However, it is likely that several of the described peptide structures may represent artifacts that are not physiologically present or degradation products from larger parent opioid structures. However, such peptide fragments could act additively or antagonize the biological response of the parent opioid, be involved in feedback control on the synthesis, release, or degradation level of the original peptide, or even act independently on a different receptor subset. Since such functions yet are poorly understood, the full physiological and pathophysiological roles of the endogenous opioids and their receptor interactions have to await further research efforts.

The purpose of this overview is to briefly summarize the present state of endogenous opioid and opiate receptor research in order to provide a basis for and a better understanding of the clinical use of opiate drugs. This chapter will focus on the distribution of endogenous opioids and on the different classes of opioid peptides and their receptors in the central nervous system. The peripheral distribution and actions of opioids have recently been reviewed elsewhere [23].

CLASSES OF ENDOGENOUS AND EXOGENOUS OPIOIDS

The term *opioid* denoting *like an opiate*, has been accepted in the terminology describing endogenous peptides and receptors related to the actions of natural products from the opium poppy or related synthetic alkaloids [21, 22]. Thus, the terms *endogenous opioid* and *opioid peptide* should be used for the wide range of gene products with affinities for the opioid receptors.

The different endogenous opioids are generated from their major precursor molecules or prohormones (table 1–1; figure 1–1). These precursors, pre-proopiomelanocortin, pre-proenkephalin, and pre-prodynorphin, in general give rise to opioid peptides belonging to the β-endorphin family, the enkephalin family, and the dynorphin family. The precursor molecules are all large molecules of a molecular size of 15,000–30,000 daltons. They are strikingly similar and are composed of approximately 260 amino acids including the signal peptides. The pre-proopiomelanocortin, pre-proenkephalin, and pre-prodynorphin molecules, which are present in low tissue concentrations, are all biologically inert, but each may produce multiple repetitive units of active opioid peptides [84, 85, 88, 89].

In addition to products belonging to these major families, opioid peptides have been identified in the brain (kyotorphin) and frog skin (dermorphin), and some may be products from hemoglobin (hemorphins) or cytochrome B (cytochrophins) (table 1–1).

Table 1–1. Described endogenous and exogenous opioids

Opioid	Alternative names and abbreviations	Amino acid sequence	Sequence reference	Nomenclature Reference
PRE-PROOPIOMELANOCORTIN products	PRE-PROOPIOCORTIN, 31 K, PRE-POMC			24,25
β-endorphin (1–31)	C-fragment, β-LPH_{61-91}	β-LPH (61–91)		
β-endorphin (1–27)	δ-endorphin	β-LPH (61–87)	26	27
β-endorphin (1–26)		β-LPH (61–86)	28	28
β-endorphin (1–18)		β-LPH (61–78)		
C'-fragment	δ-endorphin, β-LPH_{61-87}	^{61}Tyr-Gly-Gly-Phe-Met-Thr-Ser-Glu-	29	19
γ-endorphin (1–17)	β-LPH_{61-77}	Lys-Ser-Gln-Thr-Pro-Leu-Val-	29	18
α-endorphin (1–16)	β-LPH_{61-76}	^{76}Thr-^{77}Leu-Phe-Lys-Asn-Ala-Ile-Ile-Lys-Asn-Ala-^{87}His-Lys-Lys-Gly-^{91}Gln	29	30
α-N-acetyl-β-endorphin		N-acetylated BLPH (61–91)	31	31
α-N-acetyl-γ-endorphin		N-acetylated βLPH (61–77)	32	32
α-N-acetyl-α-endorphin		N-acetylated βLPH (61–76)	30	30
PRE-PROENKEPHALIN products	PRE-PROENKEPHALIN A, PRE-PROENK			33,34
[Met]enkephalin	Methionine-enkephalin-Met-enk	Tyr-Gly-Gly-Phe-Met	17	35
[Met]enkephalyl-Arg^6	pro-methionine-enkephalin, [Met]enkephalin-Arg^6	——————-Arg	35	35
[Met]enkephalyl-Lys^6	[Met]enkephalin-Lys^6	——————-Lys	36,37	36,37
[Met]enkephalyl-Arg^6-Phe^7	[Met]enkephalin-Arg^6-Phe^7, MEAP, MERF	——————-Arg-Phe	37	38
[Met]enkephalyl-Arg^6-Arg^7	[Met]enkephalin-Arg^6-Arg^7	——————-Arg-Arg	36	36,37
[Met]enkephalyl-Arg^6-Gly^7-Leu^8	[Met]enkephalin-Arg^6-Gly^7-Leu^8, MERGL	——————-Arg-Gly-Leu	39	39
Peptide F		Tyr-Gly-Gly-Phe-Met-Lys-Lys-Met-Asp-Glu-Leu-Tyr-Pro-Leu-Glu-Val-Glu-Glu-Glu-Ala-Asn-Gly-Gly-Glu-Val-Leu-Gly-Lys-Arg-Tyr-Gly-Gly-Phe-Met	40	41
Peptide I		Ser-Pro-Thr-Leu-Glu-Asp-Glu-His-Lys-Glu-Leu-Gln-Lys-Arg^{15}-Tyr-Gly-Gly-		41

Table 1–1 (continued)

Opioid	Alternative names and abbreviations	Amino acid sequence	Sequence reference	Nomenclature reference
		Phe-Met-Arg-Arg-Val-Gly-Arg-Pro-^{26}Glu-Trp-Trp-Met-Asp-TyrGln-Lys-^{34}Arg-Tyr-^{36}Gly-Gly-Phe-^{39}Leu		
Peptide E		Peptide I (15–39)	42	42
Peptide B		Phe-Ala-Glu-Pro-Leu-Pro-Ser-Glu-Glu-Glu-Gly-Glu-Ser-Tyr-Ser-Lys-Glu-Val-Pro-Glu-Met-Glu-Lys-Arg-Tyr-Gly-Gly-Phe-Met-Arg-Phe	43	44
BAM-12P		Peptide I (15–26)	44	44
BAM-20P		Peptide I (15–34)	45	45
BAM-22P		Peptide I (15–36)	45	45
Metorphamide	Adrenorphin	Peptide E (1–8) NH_2	46	46
Amidorphin		Peptide F (1–26) NH_2	47	47,49
Synenkephalin	Pre-proenkephalin (1–70)			48
[Leu]enkephalin	Leucine-enkephalin, Leu-enk	Tyr-Gly-Gly-Phe-Leu	17	17,50
PRE-PRODYNORPHIN product	PRE-PROENKEPHALIN B, PRE-PRONORPHIN			51,52
[Leu]enkephalyl-Arg^{6}	[Leu]enkephalin-Arg^{6}	Tyr-Gly-Gly-Phe-Leu-Arg	36,37,50	36,37,53
β-neo-endorphin		______-Lys-Tyr-Pro	56	56
α-neo-endorphin		______-Lys-Tyr-Pro-Lys	54	55
Dynorphin 1–8	PH-8P, Dynorphin A (1–8)	(sequence 1–8)	57	57
Dynorphin A	Dynorphin 1–17	(sequence 1–17)	58	58
Dynorphin B	Rimorphin, Dynorphin (1–13)	(sequence 20–32)	20,58,60,61	20,58,60,61
Dynorphin 32		^{1}Tyr-Gly-Gly-Phe-Leu-Arg-Arg^{8}-Ile-Arg-Pro-Lys-Leu^{13}Lys-Trp-Asp-Asn-^{17}Gln-Lys-Arg-^{20}Tyr-Gly-Gly-Phe-Leu-Arg-Arg-Gln-Phe-Lys-Val-Val^{32}Thr	59	59
Leumorphine	Dynorphin B (1–29)	Tyr-Gly-Gly-Phe-Leu-Arg-Arg-Gln-Phe-Lys-Val-Val-Thr-Arg-Ser-Gln-Glu-Asp-Pro-Asn-Ala-Tyr-Tyr-Glu-Glu-Leu-Phe-Asp-Val	51,62	62

OTHER ENDOGENOUS OPIOIDS				
Kytorphin		Tyr-Arg	63,64	63,64
Dermorphin		Tyr-D-Ala-Phe-Gly-Tyr-Pro-Ser-NH_2	65,66	65,66
Humoral endorphin	H-endorphin			67
Anodynin				68
Cytochrophin 1–4		Tyr-Pro-Phe-Thr	69	69
1–5		Tyr-Pro-Phe-Thr-Ile	69	69
Hemorphin 1–4		Tyr-Pro-Trp-Thr	70	70
1–5		Tyr-Pro-Trp-Thr-Gln	70	70
EXOGENOUS OPIOID	EXORPHINS			71
β-casomorphin (bovine)		Tyr-Pro-Phe-Pro-Gly-Pro-Ile	72,73	72,73
β-casomorphin (human)		Tyr-Pro-Phe-Val-Glu-Pro-Ile	74	74
β-casomorphin (11)		Tyr-Pro-Phe-Pro-Gly-Pro-Ile-Pro-Asn-Ser-Leu	75	75
Morphiceptin		Tyr-Pro-Phe-Pro-NH_2	76	76
OPIOID RECEPTORS				
μ (mu)			78	77
μ_1 and μ_2				78
δ (delta)				79
κ (kappa)				77
κ_1 and κ_2				80
σ (sigma)				77
ε (epsilon)				82
λ (lambda)				83

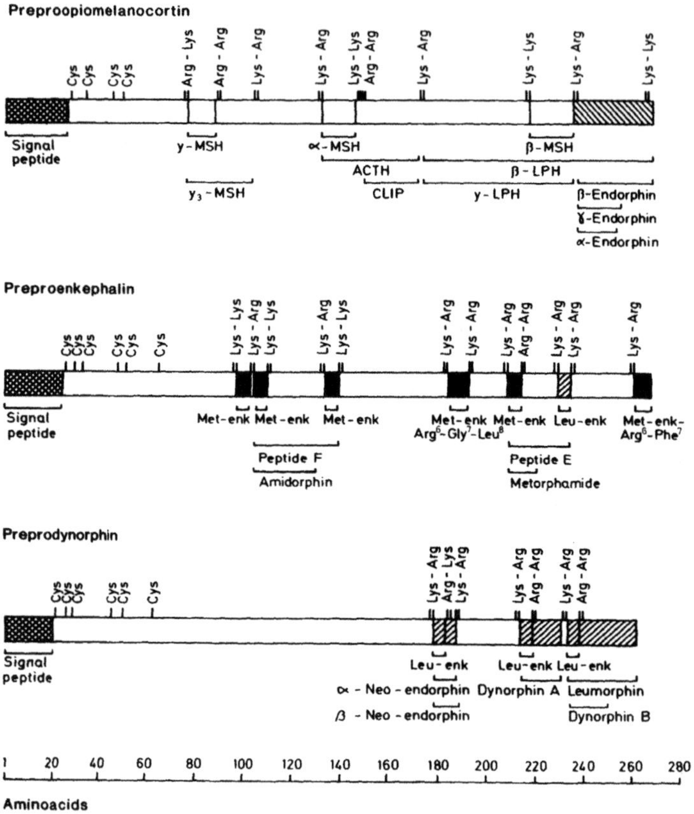

Figure 1–1. Schematic representation of the structures of the prohormones pre-proopiomelanocortin, pre-proenkephalin, and pre-prodynorphin. Indicated are the definitive and putative opioid peptides generated from each precursor molecule.

The generic term *endorphin* appeared early in the literature [4, 18] and was derived from *endo*, signifying endogenous, and *orphine*, which is a common suffix for opiates and opioids. The β-prefix for β-endorphin seemed natural when it was established that this opioid consisted of the C-fragment of β-lipotropin (β-LPH_{61-91}) [19]. The name *enkephalin*, originating from the Greek *en kephalos*, in the head, was proposed for the natural compound even before the exact structure had been elucidated [35]. Later, when two different pentapeptides with different carboxy-terminal amino acids were identified [17], they were named [Met]enkephalin and [Leu]enkephalin after their methionine and leucine residues respectively. The name *dynorphin* was originally used to describe an extraordinarily potent 13-amino-acid structure isolated from pituitary extract [20]. The name was derived from the Greek term *dynamis*, extraordinarily strong, and the suffix *orphine* used in previous opioid terminology. These names, endorphin, enkephalin, and dynorphin, have in general been used in the terminology of the newer groups of shorter of extended amino acid sequences that have appeared later in the literature [21, 22]. The extent of physiological relevance of these various structures in the different families is still widely discussed.

The pre-proopiomelanocortin is polyfunctional, containing not only the β-endorphin structure but also the sequences for ACTH and several MSH structures (figure 1–1). The β-endorphin structure has attracted most interest and most probably serves a neurotransmitter/neuromodulatory role; it may also function as neurohumoral agent [23, 84, 85]. Several truncated forms of β-endorphin have been described, like β-endorphin (1–18), β-endorphin (1–26), and β-endorphin (1–27) [28], as well as α- and γ-endorphin (table 1–1) [30]. These structures have received considerably less attention, and it is not yet known whether these peptides are primary active structures, degradation products, or artifacts. Recently, several N-acetylated endorphin structures were isolated from the pituitary gland [31, 32]. To what extent α-N-acetyl-β-endorphin, α-N-acetyl-γ-endorphin, and α-N-acetyl-α-endorphin may play any physiological or pathophysiological role still remains to be determined.

The pre-proenkephalin structure contains four repetitive Met enkephalin sequences, one [Leu]enkephalin sequence, and one sequence each of the extended [Met]enkephalin structures [Met]enkephalin-Arg^6-Gly-^{7}-Leu^8 and [Met]enkephalin-Arg^6-Phe^7 (figure 1–1). Both [Met]enkephalin and [Leu]-enkephalin no doubt serve as neurotransmitters within the control nervous system (CNS). Much interest is currently focused on the extended [Met]-enkephalin structures. These structures may serve as independent neurotransmitters/neuromodulators in the brain, gastrointestinal tract, or adrenal gland, but this hypothesis remains to be firmly established [38, 39, 86, 87].

Metorphamide and amidorphin [47, 49] and both products of pre-proenkephalin, but in contrast to other endogenous opioid peptides, both metorphamide and amidorphin possess a C-terminal amide group. Although present in high concentrations in the adrenal and/or the hypothalamic–pituitary axis, it is not clear if these two amidated opioid peptides have specific and independent physiological roles.

Pre-prodynorphin contains three repetitive [Leu]enkephalin structures; all are contained within the more extended peptide structures Neo-endorphin, Dynorphin A (1–17), Dynorphin B (20–32), or Leumorphin (figure 1–1). It is reasonable to assume that these structures all have distinct physiological roles [54, 58, 62, 85, 88].

Most of the known opioid peptides are generated from one of the three major precursor molecules by classical proteolytic cleavage at double basic amino acid residues (Arg–Arg, Arg–Lys, Lys–Arg, Lys–Lys). However, there are products from each of the three precursors that deviate from this conventional processing, where cleavage occurs at a single basic arginine residue or seemingly randomly. Thus, the products α- and γ-endorphin from pre-proopiomelanocortin as well as BAM 12 and BAM 22 from pre-proenkephalin seem to be generated by random cleavage. It is not clear whether these peptides occur naturally or if they are prevalent within the brain. From pre-prodynorphin, both Dynorphin (1–8) and Dynorphin B are generated by single Arg-residue cleavage. In contrast to α- and γ-endorphin as well as BAM 12 and 22, these dynorphin products seem to be major products from the posterior part of the pituitary or within specific neuronal tracts.

There is now evidence that all three opioid peptide precursors can generate endogenous opioid peptide structures of varying amino acid chain length. Obviously, the proteolytic processing pattern is differently regulated within different tissues, since the relative concentrations of the possible products very between these tissues [90]. Thus, not all double basic amino acid residues (Arg–Arg, Arg–Lys, Lys–Arg, Lys–Lys) seem to be equally susceptible processing sites. If all opioid precursor molecules were actually cleared at these double basic amino acid residues, the only opioid peptides generated would be β-endorphin (1–27) from pre-proopiomelanocortin [Met]enkephalin, [Leu]enkephalin, [Met]enkephalin-Arg^6-Phe^7, and [Met]enkephalin-Arg^6-Gly^7-Leu^8 from pre-proenkephalin, and [Leu]enkephalin from pre-prodynorphin. Thus, several peptides like β-endorphin (1–31), peptide E, peptide F, metorphamide, amidorphin, dynorphin A, α-neo-endorphin, and leumorphin contain one or sometimes even two intact double basic amino acid residues within their structure.

It is evident that the possible and identified cleavage products of each opioid precursor molecule differ in concentrations within different tissues. Thus, a differential processing of pre-proopiomelanocortin likely occurs within different tissues since β-endorphin (1–31) is more prominent within the anterior pituitary and hypothalamus, while the truncated forms, β-endorphin (1–26) and β-endorphin (1–27), are more prevalent in the intermediate pituitary and certain midbrain areas [90, 91]. Similarly, the longer peptides derived from pre-proenkephalin, like peptide E, peptide F, BAM 22, BAM 12, significant amounts of metorphamide, and amidorphin, are only found in the adrenal medulla [47, 49, 92, 93]. The shorter peptides [Met]enkephalin and [Leu]-enkephalin, which only exist in smaller quantities in the adrenal gland, are in contrast abundant in brain tissue. Thus the processing of pre-proenkephalin is much more complete in brain tissue than in the adrenal medulla. If the pre-prodynorphin molecule were cleaved at all sites where double basic amino acid residues were present, the only opioid peptide generated would be [Leu]-enkephalin. However, it may be possible that [Leu]enkephalin, which is present in high concentrations in many brain regions, is a product of pre-proenkephalin rather than of pre-prodynorphin. Supporting this is the fact that [Leu]enkephalin-rich brain regions are also rich in [Met]enkephalin-Arg^6-Phe^7 and [Met]enkephalin-Arg^6-Gly^7-Leu^8 rather than the extended pre-prodynorphin structures [94]. However, a considerable overlap is present. Thus, it seems like all presently known pre-prodynorphin products are the results of cleavage either at a Lys–Arg double bond or at a single Arg residue. Therefore, within cells producing dynorphin-related structures, the Arg–Arg and Arg–Lys bonds, which follow the [Leu]enkephalin structures within the pre-prodynorphin molecule, seem to be stable and untouched by the proteolytic processing enzymes in most neuronal populations in the brain. Taken together, it seems apparent that opioid peptides of different chain length can be produced not only from the different precursor molecules, but also that the processing pattern of these products is differently regulated is different tissues.

In addition to the opioid peptides originating from the defined prohormone structures, pre-proopiomelanocortin, pre-proenkephalin, and pre-prodynorphin, other opioid peptide structures have been described (table 1–1). Kyotorphin [63, 64] is a small dipeptide with analgesic properties that may induce its effects through release of other endogenous opioids. A pentapeptide precursor to kyotorphin has also been isolated from bovine brain [95]. Dermorphin [65, 66] is a heptapeptide isolated from amphibian skin. Whether these peptides are neuronally located and serve physiological roles is not yet known. The cytochrophins and hemorphins [69, 70] are peptides with opioid activity originating from mitochondrial cytochrome B and the β-, γ-, δ-, and ε-chains of hemoglobin respectively. Although analgesic, the biological relevance of these peptides remains to be established.

Exogenous opioid peptides, or exorphins, have been described in the human and other mammals. Of these peptides, the casomorphins [72–75], are generated during proteolytic cleavage of β-casein from milk products.

However, the biological relevance of the endogenous opioids that do not originate from any of the major prohormone structures, as well as the exogenous opioid structures, is not fully clarified, and further research is needed in order to gain insight to their physiological or pharmacological roles.

CENTRAL DISTRIBUTION OF ENDOGENOUS OPIOIDS

Within the brain and spinal cord, the major endogenous opioid peptide systems show a regional and distinct distribution [96–100]. Immunocytochemical and radioimmunoassay techniques have been extensively used to map neuronal networds. Some care must be taken when interpreting such data, due to the risk of cross-reactivity with peptides other than the intended antigen. However, most studies provide a reasonably consistent picture of the distribution of the various opioid peptides.

β-endorphin family

Peptides belonging to the endorphin family may be found in two separate systems: the pituitary and the extrapituitary brain tissue [101]. Within the pituitary, the highest concentrations of proopiomelanocortin products are found in the anterior and intermediate lobes [102, 103]. Both lobes contain several peptide forms, including β-endorphin and the α-N-acetylated endorphin structures [31, 32, 104, 105]. The four endorphin peptide structures that have been identified in the pituitary have also been found in several extrapituitary regions of the brain [104, 105]. In the brain, cell bodies containing peptides belonging to the endorphin family have been identified in the basal hypothalamic region and the arcuate nucleus [103, 106]. From the hypothalamic region, β-endorphin-containing neurons project to the median eminence and extend through the anterior hypothalamus to the dorsal midline thalamus. Neuronal fibers containing β-endorphinlike peptides also extend to the amygdala, preoptic area, ventral medial nuclei, paraventricular nucleus, periaqueductal gray, reticular formation, and stria terminalis [103].

Enkephalin family

Peptide structures generated from pre-proenkephalin are distinctly separated but more broadly distributed in the brain compared to β-endorphin or related peptides [103]. Peptides belonging to the enkephalin family are located in the pituitary, but in contrast to the endorphin peptides, the highest concentrations are in the posterior lobe [103, 104]. Cell bodies and fibers containing enkephalin-like immunoreactivity reside in a wide variety of regions within the brain. Thus, cell bodies are localized in the caudate nucleus, nucleus interstitials stria terminalis, central nucleus of the amygdala, paraventricular and supraoptic nuclei, perifornical region of the hypothalamus, interpeduncular nucleus, nucleus cochlearis dorsalis, nucleus vestibularis medialis, nucleus vestibularis spinalis, the central gray, reticular formation, nucleus tractus solitarius, nucleus tractus spinalis nervi trigemini, cerebellum (Golgi type II cells), olfactory bulb, olfactory tubercule, the lateral preoptic nucleus, the suprachiasmatic nucleus, cortical amygdaloid nucleus, basal amygdaloid nucleus, medial amygdaloid nucleus, hippocampus, neocortex, cingulate cortex, posterior mammilary nucleus, medial nucleus of the optic tract, brachium of the inferior colliculus, ventral tegmental nucleus, nucleus reticularis lateralis, and laminae II, III, and VII of the spinal cord. In addition, nerve cell fibers containing enkephalinlike immunoreactivity may be found in the lateral septum, the central nucleus of the amygdala, the hippocampus, cerebral cortex, corpus striatum, bed nucleus of the stria terminalis, parts of the hypothalamus, median eminence, several thalamic and subthalamic nuclei, interpeduncular nucleus, reticular formation, periaqueductal gray, parabrachial nucleus, locus coeruleus, raphe nuclei, cochlear nucleus, nucleus tractus solitarius, nucleus tractus spinalis nervi trigemini, motor nucleus of several cranial nerves, nucleus commisuralis, and substantia gelatinosa [101]. As previously pointed out, each pre-proenkephalin molecule contains four [Met]enkephalin and one [Leu]enkephalin sequences (figure 1–1). However, the ratio between [Met]enkephalin and [Leu]enkephalin is not constant from one brain region to another, and therefore it has been questioned whether the two pentapeptides might exist in the same neurons [107]. Immunohistochemical studies [97, 108] intended to separate the two enkephalins seem to indicate that [Met]enkephalin and [Leu]enkephalin sometimes occur in separate neurons. Thus, as has been discussed previously, the processing of the pre-proenkephalin molecule may differ not only between the periphery and brain tissue, but possibly also within different neuronal populations. This would provide an explanation to the occasional appearance of [Met]enkephalin and [Leu]enkephalin in separate cell groups within the brain.

Dynorphin family

The peptides that are formed by proteolytic cleavage of the pre-prodynorphin molecule, Neo-endorphin, Dynorphin A, Dynorphin B, and Leumorphine, are differently distributed within the CNS from peptides of the endorphin and enkephalin families [109, 110]. [Leu]enkephalin, however, seems to be a product of pre-prodynorphin as well as pre-proenkephalin, since the distribution of [Leu]enkephalin in some areas of the brain is similar to α-neoendorphin, Dynorphin A, or Leumorphine, while in other areas [Leu]enkephalinlike immunoreactivity is more related to pre-proenkephalin-derived peptides like [Met]enkephalin-Arg-Gly-Leu [110]. Thus, [Leu]enkephalin in the brain can be derived from either pre-proenkephalin or pre-prodynorphin, and e.g., in the striatonigral pathway, [Leu]enkephalin is derived from pre-prodynorphin-containing neurons, while in the striatopallidal pathway, [Leu]enkephalin is derived mainly from neurons containing pre-proenkephalin [110, 111]. Peptides belonging to the dynorphin family, α-neoendorphin, Dynorphin A, and Leumorphine, generally have a similar distribution pattern. The highest concentrations of pre-prodynorphin-derived peptides are found in several hypothalamic nuclei, such as the premamillary, anterior hypothalamic, and dorsomedial nuclei, and the median eminence. High concentrations are found also in other hypothalamic areas, in the area postrema, in parabracheal nuclei, and superior olive in the pons, and in nucleus tractus solitarii in the medulla oblongata. Significant amounts are detected in the dorsal and ventral horns of the spinal cord as well [112]. The distribution of the different pre-prodynorphin-derived opioids (apart from [Leu]enkephalin) was investigated in the rat and human brain [113–115]. These studies indicated that there are sometimes relatively marked differences in regional distribution. Thus, while Dynorphin B and α-neo-endorphin demonstrate a striking parallelism in distribution [116], there are major differences in the neuronal topography of Dynorphin A and Dynorphin B [113, 115]. However, Dynorphin A and α-neo-endorphin are colocalized in some neurons like, e.g., a system with the neuronal cell bodies in the head of the caudate nucleus sending nerve fibers to the substantia nigra [117]. These data strongly support the idea that differential processing of pre-prodynorphin occurs in different brain regions [115].

Opioid pathways and nociception

The control of pain by endogenous opioids is far more complex than originally thought. Basically, opioid peptides control nociception at the level of the periaqueductal gray (PAG), the medulla, and the spinal cord [8–11, 118, 119].

By the organization of the neuronal network, the different opioids from the endorphin, enkephalin, and dynorphin families may control spinal nociceptive input. The spinal modulation of nociception may involve either a *segmental control system* or a *brainstem–spinal descending control system.* The gate control theory of Melzack and Wall [120] outlined a segmental control system, by which peripheral afferent activation inhibits the transmission of the nociceptive information through second-order spinal neurons. This type of control can be elicited without supraspinal control systems but not independent of them [121]. Thus, fine-diameter afferent nerve fibers that terminate in the superficial layers of the dorsal horn not only excite second-order nociceptive neurons but also give collateral input to enkephalinlike interneurons in the same segmental region [121]. The brainstem-spinal descending system involves several levels of endogenous opioid control; the midbrain periaqueductal gray (PAG), the medullary raphe nuclei, and the dorsal horn of the spinal cord [8, 10, 11, 118, 121]. The PAG contains opioid peptides originating from all three opioid prohormone structures. In the ventrolateral and caudal portions, which have projections to the raphe nuclei, there are dense clusters of dynorphin and β-endorphin immunoreactive cells [121–123], while enkephalin cells are located more dorsally in the PAG, in a region that is a recipient of frontal cortex projections [121]. Intracerebral microinjections of β-endorphin and various enkephalin analogues, but not dynorphin [124], produce profound analgesia. Dynorphin, if anything, will antagonize analgesia produced by morphine and β-endorphin [125]. In terms of efferent pathways, the PAG seems to be an important relay station in the descending pain-modulating system. Activation of the PAG will in turn activate medullary nucleus raphe magnus neurons. The raphe neurons, which are 5-HT-containing, will send efferent information through the lateral funiculus to the nociceptive neurons of the dorsal horn of the spinal cord to yield inhibition of the nociceptive input. In addition of the descending 5-HT system, nociceptive neuronal activity is under multiple medullary controls, involving noradrenergic and other bulbospinal descending systems [10, 11, 121].

In the spinal cord, proenkephalin- and prodynorphin-derived opioid peptides may be found [121]. Enkephalin immunoreactive cells and terminals have a wide distribution in the spinal cord. Abundant enkephalin immunoreactivity may be found in the superficial dorsal horn including the marginal zone, lamine I, and laminae IIi and IIo. Some enkephalin cells are also found in laminae III, V, and VII, as well as around the central canal [126–128]. This distribution indicates actions on the nociceptive afferent and second-order neurons in laminae I, V, and VII of the spinal cord, as well as influences on nonnociceptive neurons. Compared to enkephalin, dynorphin cells and terminals are fewer in number [122, 129]. In the caudal trigeminal nucleus and dorsal horn of the spinal cord, dynorphin cells are found in laminae I and V, i.e., the location of nociceptive neurons. The presence of enkephalin- and dynorphin-related peptides in spinal cord loci associated with nociception raises the question of how and to what extent they participate in the control of pain. The hypothesis that enkephalin neurons in the dorsal horn presynaptically inhibit primary afferent fibers is not proven beyond doubt. It must also be considered that such a control might be provided by dynorphin neurons.

The segmental control system as well as the brainstem–spinal descending control system may thus employ a variety of opioid peptide inputs, and the contributions of the proopiomelanocortin-, proenkephalin, and prodynorphin-derived peptides seem to be far more complex than originally outlined.

CLASSES OF OPIOID RECEPTORS

Stereospecific binding of endogenous opioids or opiate drugs to opioid receptors is the first step in a sequence of events that leads to receptor activation and ultimately a biological response. There are strong indications that the recognition site to which the opioids bind partly constitutes a proteolipid structure, since specific binding activity decreases when brain membranes are treated with proteolytic enzymes or phospholipases [130, 131]. Although the opioid receptors still await their final isolation and purification, there are indications that the lipid modality consists of several constituents like cerebroside sulfate, phosphatidylinositol, and phosphatidylserine [13]. The cerebroside sulfate moiety seems to be of major importance, since the antinociceptive response to morphine and β-endorphin is markedly reduced in mutant, Jimpy mice with reduced brain sulfatides [132] and also after administration of antibodies to cerebroside sulfate [133]. With respect to proteins involved in opiate receptor binding, little is known. However, proteolytic enzymes like trypsin and chymotrypsin and sulfhydryl reagents markedly reduce binding to the opioid receptor [131].

There is now strong evidence that the brain contains several separate opioid receptor subtypes (tables 1–1 and 1–2). The endogenous opioid ligands produced within the brain, adrenal gland, or gastrointestinal tract are, however, not selective for any specific opioid receptor subtypes. Rather, each seems to interact with multiple receptor populations (table 1–3). However, it seems that each of the three precursors produce ligands that *predominantly* act upon one of the three main receptor subtypes, i.e., μ, δ, and κ receptors. Thus, proopiomelanocortin-derived peptides are preferentially active on the μ-receptor, proenkephalin gene-rated peptides on the δ-receptor, and opioids from prodynorphin on the κ-receptor population (table 1–3).

The concept of a heterogenous opiate receptor population was first postulated by Martin and coworkers [77] on the basis of neurophysiological and behavioral evidence in the chronic spinal dog. From studies with morphine and some benzomorphan derivatives, three different receptor subtypes were suggested, μ, κ, and σ. While later research has cast some doubt on the selectivity of some of the opiates used for receptor subclassification by Martin and colleagues, their original concept of multiple opioid receptors is supported by other models to study drugs acting on specific receptor subpopulations

Table 1–2. Opioid receptor subtypes with their proposed selective agonists and antagonists

Receptor subtype	Prototype agonist	Selective agonists	Selective antagonists	References
μ	Morphine	Tyr-D-Ala-Gly-MePhe-Glyp-ol (DAGO)	Naloxonazine (μ_1)	3,6,10,77, 82,85,90, 134,135
		Morphiceptin	β-funaltrexamine	
		Dihydromorphine	Naloxone	
σ	[Leu]enkephalin	D-Ala^2-D-Leu^5 enkephalin (DADL)	ICI 154,129	10,79,82, 85,90,134, 135
			ICI 174,864	
		D-Pen^2-D-Pen^5 enkephalin	Naloxone	
		D-Ser^2-Leu^5-enkephalin-Thr^6 (DSLET)		
ϰ	Dynorphin A and B	U 50,488	WIN-44,441–3	10,77,85, 90,134,135
		Ehtylketazocine	MR-2266	
		MR-2034	Naloxone	
ε	β-endorphin	β-endorphin	Naloxone	10,82,85, 90,134,135

U 50,488: trans-(+)-3,4-dichloro-N-methyl-[2-(1-pyrrolidinyl)cyclohexyl]-benezenacetamide methane sulphontate.
MR 2034: (−)-α-(IR,5R,9R)-5,9-dimethyl-2-(L-tetrahydrofurfuryl-2'-hydroxy-6, 7-bensomorphan.
ICI 154129: N,Nbisallyl-Tyr-Gly-Gly-ψ-(CH_2S)-Phe-Leu.
ICI 174864: N,Nbisallyl-Tyr-Aib-Aib-Phe-Leu (Aib-aminoisobutyrate).
WIN-44,441–3: (2α,6α,11S) (±)-l-cyclopentyl-5-(1,2,3,4,5,6-hexohydro-8-hydroxy-3,6,11-trimethyl-2,6-methano-3-benzazocin-ll-yl)-3-pentanone.
MR 2266: (−)-6,11α-diethyl-3-(3-purinylmethyl)-1,2,3,4,5,6-hexahydro-2,6-methano-3-benzazocin-8-ol.

[85, 134, 138]. In addition to in vivo pharmacological studies, these methods include receptor-binding assays, in vitro bioassays on isolated tissues, and studies on *selective cross-tolerance* and *selective protection* [10, 11, 85, 134, 135]. Such experiments have led to the identification or postulation of μ (mu), δ (delta), ϰ (kappa), σ (sigma), ε (epsilon), and λ (lambda) subtypes of receptors.

μ-receptor

The existence of a μ-opioid receptor was first proposed by Martin and coworkers [77] on the basis of differential pharmacological responses and lack of cross-tolerance between different opiate drugs. The μ-receptor response, characteristically elicited by morphine, included analgesia, miosis, bradycardia, hypothermia, and indifference. The existence of a specific μ-receptor site has further been substantiated by receptor-binding experiments, in vitro assays, and selective cross-tolerance and protection experiments. Although morphine still is considered as the prototype μ agonist, more specific μ-receptor agonists like DAGO, morphiceptin, and dihydromorphine (table 1–2) have been used to characterize the binding sites [134]. Such agonists are also potent in inhibiting the response to transmural stimulation in the isolated guinea pig ileum myenteric plexus-longitudinal muscle preparation, which has been shown to be rich in μ-receptors. Furthermore, in both the guinea pig

Table 1–3. Endogenous opioids as ligands on opioid receptors

Peptide	Receptor Specificity	Relative receptor afffinity			Binding affinity at preferred site K_i;nM^{-1}		
		μ	δ	κ	μ	δ	κ
Pre-proopiomelanocortin							
β-endorphin	$\mu = \delta > \varepsilon \gg \kappa$	0.52	0.46	0.02	0.49	0.42	–
Pre-proenkephalin							
[Met]enkephalin	$\delta \gg \mu$	0.09	0.91	0	–	1.10	–
[Leu]enkephalin	$\delta \gg \mu$	0.06	0.94	0	–	0.85	–
[Met]enkephalin-Arg⁶-Phe⁷	$\delta = \mu \gg \kappa$	0.60	0.36	0.04	0.29	0.18	–
[Met]enkephalin-Arg⁶-Gly⁷-Leu⁸	$\delta = \mu \gg \kappa$	0.41	0.56	0.03	0.15	0.21	–
Pre-prodynorphin							
α-neo-endorphin	$\kappa > \delta = \mu$	0.10	0.23	0.67	–	–	5.1
Dynorphin A (1–8)	$\kappa > \delta = \mu$	0.22	0.16	0.62	–	–	0.75
Dynorphin A	$\kappa \gg \mu$	0.13	0.04	0.83	–	–	8.7
Dynorphin B	$\kappa \gg \mu$	0.14	0.03	0.83	–	–	8.5

Receptor specificity, binding affinities, and relative binding affinities of the major endogenous opioids according to references 85, 136, and 137. Affinities were determined in homogenates of guinea pig brain at o°C. Affinity at the μ-site was determined with [^{3}H]-[D-Ala^2, MePhe^4, Gly-ol^5] enkephalin (1 n M), affinity at the δ-site with [^{3}H]-[D-Ala^2, D-Leu^5] enkephalin (1 n M), and affinity at the κ-site with [^{3}H]-(−)-bremazocine after suppression of residual μ- and δ-binding. Inhibition constant: $IC_{50}/(1+[L]/K_D)$; affinity constant: K_i;nM^{-1}; relative affinity: K_i^{-1} for μ, δ or κ/[(K_i^{-1} for μ)+(K_i^{-1} for δ)+(K_i^{-1} for κ)].

ileum (μ- and κ-receptors) and the mouse vas deferens (μ-, δ-, and κ-receptors), long-term treatment with μ-selective opiates like sufentanil renders the tissue tolerant to other μ-agonists but not to δ- or κ-receptor activating agents [85, 134]. Additionally, when selective opioid receptor agonists are used in an in vitro preparation together with an irreversible nonselective opioid receptor antagonist like β-chlornaltrexamine (β-CNA), the specific agonist will protect the receptors from the irreversible ligand, and sensitivity to the selective agonist or other agents acting on the same receptor subtype (e.g., μ-receptors) will be retained [85, 134].

At the subcellular level, activation of μ-receptors is associated with an increase in (K^+) conductance [141]. It is also possible that the μ-receptor could be functionally coupled to adenylatecyclase [134].

Among the endogenous opioid peptides, there is no structure highly selective for μ-opioid receptors (table 1–3). However, most data indicate that β-endorphin and to some extent also the extended [Met]enkephalin-Arg^6-Gly^7-Leu^8, but not the enkephalin pentapeptides or prodynorphin products, will interact with the μ-receptors. Although the peripheral in vitro bioassay systems could differentiate between μ- and δ-receptors, they could not explain other in vivo effects like complex interactions between morphine (μ) and enkephalin (predominantly δ) analgesia. On the basis of cross-tolerance experiments and the finding of a novel high-affinity opiate-binding site in the brain, Pasternak and coworkers [139] have offered another explanation. They postulate that both morphine and the enkephalins are involved in a common receptor mechanism. Both agents could apparently bind and share a high-affinity (μ_1) site, while for low-affinity binding, morphinelike drugs are bound to a μ_2-site and enkephalins to a δ-site. This three-site model implies that the supraspinal analgesia after morphine, β-endorphin, or enkephalin is mediated largely through high-affinity μ_1-binding sites, whereas spinal analgesia involves δ-site, and effects like respiratory depression and bradycardia are due to interaction with low-affinity μ_2-binding sites.

δ-receptor

As previously outlined, several peripheral in vitro bioassay systems were used to differentiate between opiate receptor subtypes. In experiments on two isolated tissue preparations, the guinea pig ileum (μ and κ) and the mouse vas deferens (μ, δ, and κ), Kosterlitz's group in Aberdeen [79] found major differences between the enkephalins and morphine. They postulated a receptor type, the δ-receptor, that was more selective for the enkephalins than for morphine, which was preferentially μ-selective. Further evidence for a δ-receptor was found through testing more δ-receptor-enriched preparations like the hamster vas deferens [85] and by demonstration of an extensive cross-tolerance to δ-agonists but not to μ-agonists in peripheral bioassays [140]. Binding studies in brain homogenates also confirmed the existence of separate selective morphine (μ) and enkephalin (δ) sites [79]. Additionally, in μ-receptor-tolerant mouse vas deferens preparations, there was no tolerance to δ-agonists and vice versa. Chronic exposure to D-Ala^2-D-Leu^5-enkephalin (DADL; δ-agonist) produced selective tolerance to the δ-agonist [Leu]enkephalin but not the μ-agonist normorphine.

δ-receptors have, like μ-receptors, been coupled to (K^+) conductance, but, unlike the μ-receptor, the δ-receptor does not seem to be coupled to adenylate cyclase [134, 141].

Apart from the prototype δ-agonist [Leu]enkephalin, more selective modified peptide structures, like D-Ala^2-D-Leu^5 enkephalin (DADL), D-Pen^2-D-Pen^5-enkephalin, and D-Ser^2-Leu^5-enkephalin-Thr^6 (DSLET), have been synthesized and tested (table 1–2). ICI 154,129 and ICI 174,864 represent two highly selective δ-receptor antagonists with virtually no effects on the μ- and κ-receptors, and have been used in the in vivo discrimination of δ-receptors. The most selective of the endogenous opioids that bind to the δ-receptor are [Met]enkephalin and [Leu]enkephalin (table 1–3). [Met]enkephalin has a somewhat higher affinity for the δ-receptor than [Leu]enkephalin. The more extended proenkephalin structures [Met]enkephalin-Arg^6-Phe^7 and [Met]-enkephalin-Arg^6-Gly^7-Leu^8 have approximately equal relative affinity for δ- and μ- receptors, but the binding affinity at the preferred site is lower compared to the enkephalin pentapeptides (table 1–3). Some of the prodynorphin split products, like α-neo-endorphin and Dynorphin A (1–8), demonstrate some affinity for the δ-receptor site as well.

ϰ-receptor

Originally, Martin and coworkers also postulated a ϰ-receptor [77]. Durgs like ketocyclazocine and ethlketocyclazocine (ethylketazocine) reduced responses to noxious stimuli, caused sedation, had greater spinal than supraspinal antinociceptive effects in the chronic spinal dog, and were proposed as ϰ-agonists. Furthermore, these drugs did not substitute for morphine in μ-receptor-dependent animals, caused less physical dependence, and had a withdrawal syndrome distinct from morphine. Further evidence for a putative ϰ-receptor was demonstrated in in vivo bioassay systems. Several proposed ϰ-agonists were found to be relatively more potent in the guinea pig ileum (μ and ϰ) assay than in the mouse vas deferens (μ, δ, and ϰ) assay as compared with a variety of other opiate drugs [6, 79, 85]. Potent effects of ϰ-agonists can also be demonstrated in the rabbit vas deferens preparation, which has only opioid receptors of the ϰ-receptor subtype [142]. In the guinea pig ileum preparation, selective tolerance can be demonstrated for μ- and ϰ-agonists [143]. Selective protection experiments were performed in guinea pig brain membranes by Goldstein and coworkers [144, 145]. They demonstrated that with the irreversible antagonist, β-chlornaltrexamine, ϰ- but not μ-opioid receptor sites are protected against inactivation when the tissue is exposed to dynorphin A (1–8) or dynorphin A (1–17). In contrast, sufentanyl preserved the function of μ- but not ϰ-receptors. Demonstrating ϰ-sites through binding studies in the brain proved more difficult owing to the ability of ϰ-drugs to bind to a number of other receptor classes [6, 135]. However, subsequent selective protection experiments provided sufficient proof of ϰ-receptor binding in the CNS [135]. A subclassification of ϰ-receptors into $\varkappa_1$- and $\varkappa_2$-binding sites was recently suggested on the basis of studies on the binding characteristics of [^{3}H]-etorphine in guinea pig striatum and lumbosacral spinal cord [80, 81]. In the striatum and in the spinal cord, [^{3}H]ethylketo-cyclazocine interacted with two components, a high- and a low-affinity site, in contrast to [^{3}H]-etorphine, which only interacted with the high-affinity site. Dynorphin (1–17) was suggested to interact with the low-affinity $\varkappa_1$-binding site, while [Met]enkephalin was a potent ligand for the high-affinity $\varkappa_2$-binding site.

At the membrane level, activation of ϰ-receptors causes a quite different effect than μ- and δ-receptor activation; voltage-dependent [Ca^{++}] conductance is reduced, leading to a reduced [Ca^{++}] entry into the cell [141]. Although it is not known whether μ- and δ-receptors coexist on the same neuron, data indicate that opioid receptors of the ϰ-type can coexist with μ- and δ-receptors [141].

Dynorphin A and B are regarded as the prototype ϰ-agonists (table 1–2) with high selectivity as well as binding affinity to the ϰ-site (table 1–3). Other prodynorphin fragments like Dynorphin A (1–8) and α-neo-endorphin also have high affinity for the κ-opioid receptor subtype. However, Dynorphin A (1–8) and α-neo-endorphin are considerably less potent compared to Dynorphin A and B (table 1–3).

ε-receptor

A separate ε-opiate receptor has been proposed on the basis of experiments on the rat vas deferens [82]. On this specific preparation, the responses to electrical stimulation are blocked by β-endorphin, and it was thought that the rat vas deferens was a suitable preparation for μ-receptors. However, in this specific preparation morphine and μ-specific stable enkephalin analogues have no effect [146]. Furthermore, there are no indications of δ- or κ-receptor activity [85] except that κ-agonists seem to antagonize the action of β-endorphin in this specific tissue preparation [138]. Therefore, in the rat vas deferens, μ-receptors may coexist with a putative unique ε-receptor for which β-endorphin has an unusually high affinity [82, 85]. However, to establish this β-endorphin binding site as a true opioid receptor subtype, specific binding cross-tolerance as well as protection experiments need to be performed.

σ-receptor

In their original subclassification of receptors, Martin and coworkers [77] suggested the existence of a unique opiate receptor classified as σ. Interaction with this receptor was not associated with antinociception but rather with mydriasis, tachycardia, and mania. A typical agonist on the σ-receptor was N-allyl-norcyclazocine (SKF 10.047), and interaction with the σ-receptor was associated with the psychotomimetic actions of many opiate derivatives. However, prototypic σ-agonists like SKF 10.047 are not selective but exhibit potent high affinity for μ-receptors as well [134]. The low-affinity σ-site can be blocked by phenylcyclidine (PCP) [147], a psychotomimetic drug, and therefore the proposed σ-receptor may be a composite μ–PCP binding site and not a true opioid receptor.

λ-receptor

The λ-site is a postulated high-affinity site for 4,5-epoxymorphinans. This site was described by Grevel and Sadee [83] based on the finding the diprenorphine, which has affinity to μ-, δ-, and κ-receptors, failed to completely displace ^{3}H-naloxone in vitro and in vivo. This indicated a nonconventional site that could be distinguished from the μ-binding site be relative lability and a differential CNS distribution. Thus, in the cerebellum where low μ-receptor binding is found, the λ-binding was among the highest found in the brain [83].

The concept of opioid receptor subtyping is now firmly established, and at present in vitro and in vivo model favor the existence of μ-, δ-, and κ-opioid binding sites. The ε-receptor may exist as a separate entity, while σ- as well as λ-opioid-receptor binding sites are not convincingly supported by data to enable us to grade them as true opioid-receptor subtypes. It is still unresolved whether the major opioid-receptor subtypes, μ-, δ-, κ-sites, are distinct proteolipid structures of different molecular weights, or if they represent interconvertible forms of the same molecular structure. Regarding the molecular basis for the interconvertible theory, it is hypothesized that the various receptor subtypes are of the same polypeptide species on different lipid or membrane environments, are in different conformational or aggregational states, or exist in the presence or absence of small effector regulatory molecules [134]. However, this issue will only be ultimately solved with the solubilization, purification, characterization, and sequencing of all the different forms of opioid receptor subtypes.

CENTRAL DISTRIBUTION OF OPIOID RECEPTORS

It is a general finding when comparing endogenous opioid peptides and opioid receptor distributions that areas that contain the largest amounts of opioid ligands contain the highest density of opioid binding sites as well. This finding indeed provides strong evidence for the idea that the endogenous opioid peptides are neurotransmitters acting locally at specific binding sites. However, a specific binding site must elicit a specific physiological or pharmacological response in order to provide a full insight into the mechanisms underlying the observed effects of a class of agents, regardless of whether those agents are administered exogenously or released endogenously from a nerve terminal in the specific region.

Using autoradiographic techniques, each of the major receptor subtypes in the brain, μ, δ, and κ, have been mapped out [10, 11, 148–157]. In the rat and the primate, a high density of total [^{3}H]-opioid binding is found in the striatum, and especially in the caudate and putamen. High and significant densities of binding are also found in the medial part of the thalamus and in the posterior and lateral parts of the hypothalamus. Several parts of the mesencephalon, like the interpeduncular nucleus, central gray, and reticular formation, exhibit high opioid binding, as well as the lateral parabracheal region of the pons and the nucleus tractus solitarius and nucleus ambiquus of the medulla oblongata. In the spinal cord, the highest density of [^{3}H]-opioid binding sites is found in lamina I, II, and III of the dorsal horn [13–15, 152]. Cortical regions of the primate generally demonstrate a low density of binding compared to the subcortical areas. In the thalamus and hypothalamus, there are higher concentrations of μ- than σ- and κ-receptors, and in the striatum the μ-receptors appear in clusters while δ-receptors occur in a more diffusely organized pattern [158, 159]. The δ-receptor is more prominent in limbic structures and in some areas of the pons and medulla oblongata [151, 158]. The most selective localization of κ-receptors occurs in the deep layers of lamina V and VI of the cerebral cortex and also, to some extent, in striatal regions of the brain [149, 153, 158, 159]. The high density of total opioid receptor binding found in lamina, I, II, and III of the dorsal horn in the spinal cord [15, 152] consists of μ-, δ- as well as κ-opioid binding sites [10, 11, 81, 158, 160]. Extrapolation of the opioid receptor distribution patterns obtained in animals to humans must, however, be made with caution; there is great variation between species. This may be particularly demonstrated in the cerebellum, where binding sites are predominantly of the μ-type in the humans. The rabbit cerebellum has binding sites of the μ-opioid type as well, while in the guinea pig cerebellum, almost all binding sites are of the κ-type. In this species, as in the mouse and rat, almost no μ-receptors can be identified [85].

OPIOID RECEPTORS IN ANALGESIA

Experimental as well as clinical studies show that the tested putative μ-, κ-, and ε-agonists all induce potent analgesia [12, 156]. Injections of μ-agonists such as morphine, fentanyl, methadone, meperidine, and etorphine in the region of PAG elicit profound analgesia [7, 161–163]. More selective δ-agonists like D-Ala^2-Met-enkepalinamide [164] as well as agonists on the ε-receptor like β-endorphin [165] also induce analgesia by PAG injections. In contrast to the potent analgetic effects of μ-, δ-, and ε-agonists in the PAG, κ-agonists like etylketocyklazocine are inactive and do not elicit analgesia after microinjections into the PAG [166]. At the spinal level, μ- and δ-agonists possess potent analgesic activity. Thus μ-agonists such as morphine, fentanyl, sufentanil, lofentanil, alfentanil, and methadone all induce antinociception or analgesia in subprimate and primate models [12]. These agents have all been used also in cancer as well as postoperative pain treatment in the human [167]. Several δ-agonists such as DADL and DSLET, but not the naturally occurring pentapeptides [Met]enkephalin or [Leu]enkephalin, possess strong antinociceptive actions [12] upon spinal application. DADL has been given to man [168, 169], where a potent analgesic affect was observed without cross-tolerance to μ-opioid agonists like morphine. In contrast, the μ-, δ-, and ε-agonist β-endorphin demonstrates partial cross-tolerance to morphine in animals rendered tolerant to β-endorphin by repeated intrathecal or systemic injections [12]. While μ- and δ-opioid receptor agonists exhibit potent antinociceptive effects in animals, as measured by cutaneous thermal measures like the tail flick and hot plate tests, κ-opioid-receptor agonists are generally insensitive in these tests [12, 170–172]. In contrast, when tested in visceral chemical tests like the writhing test, κ-agonists like U 50488 showed significant activity [12]. In this test, μ-opioid agonists like morphine but not δ-ligands like DADL demonstrated an antinociceptive potential [12]. Most data indicate that there are no major differences between the rodent and primate models employed and man in terms of receptor subpopulations and modulation of spinal nociception. Nevertheless, there may still be differences between species due to type of pain or consequence of pharmacokinetic reasons when opioid or opiate analgesics are administered by the spinal route.

Thus, on the spinal level, there are three different opioid receptor subpopulations that, when activated, will lead to selective modulation of the response to noxious stimuli. Furthermore, the action of μ- and δ-agonists on the cutaneous thermal responses and μ- and κ-agonists on chemical visceral responses indicates differential coding of spinal afferents through which the stimuli are transmitted.

RECEPTOR BINDING PROFILES AND PHARMACOLOGY OF OPIATE DRUGS

Naturally occuring or synthetic substances like morphine and its derivatives were known not only to induce analgesia but also to interact with specific receptors long before the endogenous opioid peptides were known [1, 6]. The molecular shape permitted these foreign compounds to act as drugs by fitting into the various receptor subtypes of the endogenous compounds that played normal role in human and animal physiology and pathophysiology. Indeed, the rigid structural requirements for opiate drug action, stereospecificity, and the existence of agonists as well as antagonists suggested the existence of receptor structures with specific binding characteristics that could be activated by the endogenous peptides and by the various opiate drugs. However, comparing the molecular shape of the endogenous opioid peptides and synthetic opiates has not yet resulted in any increased knowledge of the receptor structures. One of the main reasons for this is that opioids, especially the small enkephalin peptides, are very flexible molecules that may adopt several different configurations. However, the conformations that the enkephalins prefer in soild state or in solution seem to be little correlated to the conformation adopted at the receptor [173]. In spite of this, it can be claimed that the conformation that the enkephalin as well as other opioids adopt at the receptor is not energetically disfavored solution conformation. However, although the endogenous opioids have been of little or no use in guiding the synthesis of new opiate drugs, today we have access to both relatively specific agonists and antagonists at the major opioid receptor subtypes (table 1–2). These agents have been used to characterize the receptor profiles of current clinically available opiate analgesics. In table 1–4, the effects of the major opiates are given on the μ-, δ, κ-, *and* σ-opioid-receptor subtypes. The prototype μ-agonist is morphine but also fentanyl, and its newer derivatives are selective and highly potent μ-agonists [12]. Buprenorphine also seems to be highly selective for the μ-receptor subtype [174]. The partial μ-agonists are clearly agonists at the receptor in small doses, but at higher doses they possess competitive antagonistic effects, which apparently result from their slow rate of dissociation from the μ-receptor [135]. This seems to be the cause of their ceiling effect in analgesic activity. The agonist/antagonist analgesics all possess multiple receptor affinities that generally include μ-antagonism, κ-agonism, and σ-agonism. This spectrum of receptor interaction is responsible not only for their analgesic effects but for their side effects as well, especially the psychotomimetic dose-limiting problems seen with these drugs [135]. The mechanism by which many analgesics exert their antinociceptive and behavioral effects is often complex and poorly understood. For many drugs, the analgesic effect is mediated by μ- as well as κ-receptors, both of which elicit naloxone-

Table 1–4. Agonist–antagonist actions of opiate anaglesics on opioid receptor subtypes

Opiate drug	Receptor subtype			
	μ	δ	ϰ	σ
Agonists				
Morphine	Ag	O	(Ag)	O
Oxymorphone	Ag	(Ag)	pAg	–
Levorphanol	Ag	O	pAg	–
Codeine*	Ag	O	(Ag)	–
Heroin* (diacetylmorphine)	Ag	O	(Ag)	–
Etorphine	Ag	Ag	Ag	–
Methadone	Ag	O	(Ag)	–
Pethidine (meperidine)	Ag	O	Ag	–
Meptazinol	Ag (μ_1)	O	O	–
Fentanyl	Ag	(Ag)	(Ag)	–
Sufentanil	Ag	–	–	–
Lofentanil	Ag	–	–	–
Partial agonists				
Buprenorphine	pAg	(Ag)	O	O
Propiram	pAg	–	–	O
Agonists/antagonists				
Butorphanol	(Ant)	–	Ag	Ag
Nalbuphine	Ant	–	pAg	Ag
Pentazocine	Ant	pAg	Ag	Ag
Antagonists				
Nalorphine	Ant	pAg	pAg	Ag
Naloxone	Ant	Ant	Ant	O

Summary of the qualitative actions of opiate drugs based on in vitro receptor-binding isolated tissue experiments as well as in vivo pharmacology in animals and man [1, 12, 135 ,174]. Ag = agonist; Ant = competitive antagonist; pAg = partial agonist; O = no significant action; – = not yet fully studied; () = weak effect.
* Both codeine and heroine act as prodrugs. Codeine (methylmorphine) is coverted to morphine (to approximately 10%) and heroin (diacetylmorphine) is rapidly converted to monoacetylmorphine and morphine, both of which are active on opioid receptors.

sensitive alagesia. However, unlike the μ-agonists, ϰ-agonists do not suppress abstinence reactions in animals rendered tolerant to morphine, and they do not exhibit cross-tolerance with morphine [135].

Evidently, in terms of selectivity, most endogenous opioids (table 1–3) as well as opiate analgesics (table 1–4) are not selective for one specific subtype of opioid receptor but exert their actions through multiple receptors. This may indicate that the different opioid receptor structures, at least the μ-, δ-, and ϰ-sites, are relatively similar and perhaps developed late during evolution. Therefore, even slight changes in molecular structure of the opioid peptides or opiate alkaloids may result in marked changes in the binding profile of the ligand. However, structural molecular changes may alter lipophilicity–hydrophilicity, pKa, and susceptibility to metabolic degradation, and therefore the physiological and pharmacological effects of various agents may also differ due to pharmacokinetic reasons [167, 175].

CONCLUSIONS

Since the first discovery of the endogenous opioids in 1975, research has revealed a remarkable complexity of not only the endogenous opioid peptide ligands but also of their interactions with multiple subpopulations of opioid receptors. The different prohormones — proopiomelanocortin, proenkephalin, and prodynorphin — give rise to a variety of active peptide structures of the endorphin, enkephalin, and dynorphin families. Processing of the prohormone structures may occur differently in the periphery and the central nervous system as well as between different areas or nerve tracts within the brain. Several subpopulations of opioid receptors have been identified or proposed, and among the four major classes — μ-, δ-, κ-, and ε-receptors — β-endorphin seems to interact with μ-, δ-, and ε-receptors, [Met]enkephalin and [Leu]-enkephalin almost exclusively with δ-receptors, and Dynorphin A, Dynorphin B, and α-neo-endorphin with κ-receptors and to some extent also with μ- and δ-sites.

Endogenous pain control may involve a segmental action at the spinal cord level or effects through a brainstem–spinal descending control system. At the level of the spinal cord, activation of μ-, δ-, and κ-receptors results in an inhibition of cutaneous thermal and/or visceral chemical stimuli. At the level of the periaqueductal gray, μ- and δ- but not κ-receptor activation results in antinociception.

Synthetic compounds are available that bind almost exclusively to one receptor site, but several clinically used drugs demonstrate interactions with more than one opioid receptor subtype.

Within the opioid system it seems likely that the various receptor subpopulations are of greater importance to determine the physiological or pharmacological action than the endogenous peptide ligands, since these lack selectivity. It may therefore be predicted that for the future development of the opioid and opiate area, the most important achievement will be the synthesis and development of agonists and antagonists highly selective for on receptor subtype. This will presumably lead to improvements in the treatment of a variety of diseases, as we have seen for the adrenergic and histaminergic areas over the past decades.

REFERENCES

1. Jaffe JH, Martin WR. 1985. Opioid analgesics and antagonists. In Goodman-Gilman A, Goodman LS, Rall TW, Murad F (eds): The Pharmacological Basis of Therapeutics. New York: MacMillan Publishing Co., pp. 491–531.
2. Langley JN. 1901. Observations on the physiological action of extracts of the supra-renal bodies. J Physiol (Lond) 27:237–256.
3. Pert CB, Snyder SH. 1973. Opiate receptor: Demonstration in nervous tissue. Science 179:1011–1014.
4. Simon EJ, Hiller JM, Edelman I. 1973. Stereospecific binding of the potent narcotic analgesic [^{3}H] etorphine to rat brain homogenates. Proc Natl Acad Sci USA 70:1947–1949.
5. Terenius L. 1973. Stereospecific interaction between narcotic analgesics and a synpatic plasma membrane fraction of rat cerebral cortex. Acta Pharmacol Toxicol 32:317–320.

6. Goodman RR, Pasternak GW. 1984. Multiple opiate receptors. In Kuhar M, Pasternak G (eds): Analgesics: Neurochemical, Behavioral and Clinical Perspectives. New York: Raven Press, pp. 69–96.
7. Tsou K, Jang CS. 1964. Studies on the site of analgesic action of morphine by intracerebral micro-injection. Scientia Sinica 13:1–25.
8. Yaksh T. 1981. Spinal opiate analgesia. Characteristics and principles of action. Pain 11: 293–346.
9. Yaksh T, Hammond D. 1982. Peripheral and central substrates involved in rostrad transmission of nociceptive information. Pain 13:1–85.
10. Yaksh T. 1984. Multiple opioid receptor systems in brain and spinal cord: Part 1. Eur J Anaesthesiol 1:171–199.
11. Yaksh T. 1984. Multiple opioid receptor systems in brain and spinal cord: Part 2. Eur J Anaesthesiol 1:201–243.
12. Yaksh TL, Noueihed R. 1985. The physiology and pharmacology of spinal opiates. Annu Rev Pharmacol Toxicol 25:433–462.
13. Atweh SF, Kuhar MJ. 1977. Autoradiographic localization of opiate receptors in rat brain. I. Spinal cord and lower medulla. Brain Res 124:53–67.
14. Atweh SF, Kuhar MJ. 1977. Autoradiographic localization of opiate receptors in rat brain. II. The brain stem. Brain Res 129:1–12.
15. Atweh SF, Kuhar MJ. 1977. Autoradiographic localization of opiate receptors in rat brain. III. The telencephalon. Brain Res 134:393–405.
16. Terenius L, Wahlström, A. 1975. Search for an endogenous ligand for the opiate receptor. Acta Physiol Scand 94:74–81.
17. Hughes J, Smith TW, Kosterlitz HW, Fothergill LA, Morgan BA, Morris HR. 1975. Identification of two related pentapeptides from the brain with potent opiate agonist activity. Nature (Lond) 258:577–579.
18. Bradbury AF, Smyth DG, Snell CR, Birdsall NJM, Hulme EC. 1976. C fragment of lipotropin has a high affinity for brain opiate receptors. Nature (Lond) 260:793–795.
19. Li CH, Chung D. 1976. Isolation and structure of an untriakontapeptide with opiate activity from camel pituitary glands. Proc Natl Acad Sci USA 73:1145–1148.
20. Goldstein A, Tachibana S, Lowney LI, Hunkapiller M, Hood L. 1979. Dynorphin (1–13), an extraordinarily potent opioid peptide. Proc Natl Acad Sci USA 76:6666–6671.
21. Kitchen I. 1984. The rise and fall of endogenous opioid nomenclature. Prog Neurobiol 22:345–358.
22. Kitchen I. 1985. Endogenous opioid nomenclature: Light at the end of the tunnel. Gen Pharmac 16:79–84.
23. Hedner T, Cassuto J. 1987. Opioids and opioid receptors in peripheral tissues. Scand J Gastroenterol 22 (Suppl. 130), 27–46.
24. Rubenstein M, Stein S, Udenfriend S. 1978. Characterisation of pro-opiocortin, a new precursor to opioids peptides and corticotropin. Proc Natl Acad Sci USA 75:669–672.
25. Chretien M, Bejannet S, Gossard F, Gianoulakis C, Crine P, Lis M, Seidah NG. 1979. From β-lipotropin to β-endorphin and "pro-opio-melanocortin". Can J Biochem 57:1111–1121.
26. Li C, Barnafi L, Chretien M, Chung D. 1965. Isolation and amino acid sequence of β-LPH from sheep pituitary gland. Nature (Lond) 208:1093–1094.
27. Bradbury AF, Smyth DG, Snell CR. 1976. Prohormones of β-melanotropin (β-melanoctye-stimulating hormone, β-MSH) and corticotropin (adrenocorticotropic hormone, ACTH): Structure and activation. In Polypeptide hormones: Molecular and Cellular Aspects. CIBA Foundation Symposium. North Holland: Elsevier/Excerpta Medica, pp. 61–75.
28. Vuolteenaho O. 1984. Beta-endorphin-related peptides in the human pituitary. Isolation and characterization of major immunoreactive peptides, including the formerly unrecognized peptide beta-endorphin 1–18. Acta Physiol Scand (Suppl) 531:1–84.
29. Nakanishi S, Inoue A, Kita T, Nakamurza M, Change ACY, Cohen SN, Numa S. 1979. Nucleotide sequence of cloned cDNA for bovine corticotropin-β-lipotropin precursor. Nature (Lond) 278:423–427.
30. Ling N, Burgus R, Guillemin R. 1976. Isolation, primary structure and synthesis of α and γ endorphin, two peptides of hypothalamic–hypophysical origin with morphinomimetic activity. Proc Natl Acad Sci USA 73:3942–3946.
31. Smith AI, Cheng MC, Funder JW. 1985. The identification and characterization of

α-N-acetylated β-endorphin in the human pituitary gland. FEBS Lett 185:109–111.
32. Barbach JPH, van Tol HHM, Wiegant WH, van Ooijen RA, Maes RAA. 1985. Identification of Nα-acetyl-α-endorphin and Nα-acetyl-γ-endorphin isolated from the neurointermediate lobe of the rat pituitary gland. J Biol Chem 260:6663–6669.
33. Noda M, Furutani Y, Takahashi H, Toyosato M, Hirose T, Inayama S, Nakanishi S, Numa S. 1982. Cloning and sequence analysis of cDNA for bovine adrenal preproenkephalin. Nature (Lond) 295:202–206.
34. Gubler U, Seeburg P, Hoffman BJ, Gage LP, Udenfriend S. 1982. Molecular cloning establishes proenkephalin as precursor of enkephalin containing peptides. Nature (Lond) 295:206–208.
35. Huang W-Y, Chang RCC, Kastin AJ, Coy DH, Schally AV. 1979. Isolation and structure of pro-methionine-enkephalin: Potential enkephalin precursor from porcine hypothalamus. Proc Natl Acad Sci USA 76:6177–6180.
36. Lewis RV, Stern AS, Kimura S. Rossier J, Stein S. Udenfriend S. 1980. An about 50.000-Dalton protein in adrenal medulla. A common precursor of Met- and Leu-eukephalin. Science 208:1459–1461.
37. Stern AS, Lewis RV, Kimura S, Rossier J, Stein S, Udenfriend S. 1980. Opioid hexapeptides and heptapeptides in adrenal medulla and brain — Possible implications on the biosynthesis of enkephalins. Arch Biochem Biophys 205:606–613.
38. Stern AS, Lewis RV, Kimura S, Rossier J, Gerbier LD, Brink L, Stern S, Udenfriend S. 1979. Isolation of the opioid heptapeptide Met-enkephalin (Arg^6, Phe^7) from bovine adrenal medullary granules and striatum. Proc Natl Acad Sci USA 76:6680–6683.
39. Kilpatrick DL, Jones, BN, Kojima K, Udenfriend S. 1981. Identification of the octapeptide [Met]enkephalin-Arg^6-Gly^7-Leu^8 in extracts of bovine adrenal medulla. Biochem Biophys Res Comm 103:698–705.
40. Jones BN, Stern AS. Lewis RV, Kimura S, Stein S. Udenfriend S, Shively JE. 1980. Structure of 2 adrenal polypeptides containing multiple enkephalin sequences. Arch Biochem Biophys 240:392–395.
41. Kimura S, Lewis RV, Stern AS, Rossier J, Stein S, Udenfriend S. 1980. Probable precursors of leu-enkephalin and metenkephalin in adrenal medulla: Peptides of 3–5 kilodaltons. Proc Natl Acad Sci USA 77:1681–1685.
42. Kilpatrick DL, Taniguchi T, Jones BN, Stern AS, Shively JE, Hullihan J, Kimura S, Stein S. Udenfriend S. 1981. A highly potent 3200-Dalton adrenal opioid peptide that contains both a [Met]- and [Leu]-enkephalin sequence. Proc Natl Acad Sci USA 78:3265–3268.
43. Stern AS, Jones BN, Shively JE, Stein S, Udenfriend S. 1981. Two adrenal opioid polypeptides: Proposed intermediates in the processing of proenkephalin. Proc Natl Acad Sci USA 78:1962–1966.
44. Mizuno K, Minamino N, Kangawa K, Matsuo H. 1980. A new endogenous opioid peptide from bovine adrenal medulla: Isolation and amino acid sequence of a dodecapeptide (BAM-12P). Biochem Biophys Res Comm 95:1482–1488.
45. Mizuno K, Minamino N, Kangawa K, Matsuo H. 1980. A new family of endogenous "big" met-enkephalins from bovine adrenal medulla: Purification and structure of docosa (BMA-22P) and eicosapeptide (BAM-20P) with very potent opiate activity. Biochem Biophys Res Comm 97:1283–1290.
46. Weber E, Esch FS, Bohlen P, Paterson S, Corbett AD, McKnight AT, Kosterlitz HW, Barchas JD, Evans CJ. 1983. Metorphamide: Isolation, structure and biologic activity of an amidated opioid octapeptide from bovine brain. Proc Natl Acad Sci USA 80:7362–7373.
47. Matsuo H, Miyata A, Mizuno K. 1983. Novel C-terminally amidated opioid peptide in human phaeochromacytoma tumour. Nature 305:721–723.
48. Liston DR. Vanderhaeghen JJ, Rossier J. 1983. Presence in brain of synenkephalin, a proenkephalin immunoreactive protein which does not contain enkephalin. Nature 302:62–65.
49. Seizinger BR, Liebich DC, Gramsch C, Herz A. Weber E, Evans CJ, Esch FS, Böhlen P. 1985. Isolation and structure of a novel C-terminally amidated opioid peptide, amidorphin, from bovine adrenal medulla. Nature 313:57–59.
50. Kosterlitz HW, Hughes J. 1975. Some thoughts on the significance of enkephalin, the endogenous ligand. Life Sci 17:91–96.
51. Kakidani H, Furutani Y, Takahashi H, Noda M, Morimoto Y, Hirose T, Asai M, Inayama S, Nakanishi S, Numa S. 1982. Cloning and sequence analysis of cDNA for porcine β-neo-

endorphin/dynorphin precursor. Nature (Lond) 298:245–249.
52. Rossier J. 1982. Opioid peptides have found their roots. Nature (Lond) 298:221–222.
53. Kangawa K, Mizuno K, Minamino N, Matsuo H. 1980. Radioimmunoassay for detecting pro-leu-enkephalins in tissue extracts: Purification and identification of Arg^6 leu-enkephalin in porcine pituitary. Biochem Biophys Res Comm 95:1467–1474.
54. Kangawa K, Minamino N, Chino N, Sakakibara S, Matsuo H. 1981. The complete amino acid sequence of the α-neo-endorphin. Biochem Biophys Res Comm 99-871-878.
55. Kangawa K, Matsuo H. 1979. α-neo-endorphin: A "big" leu-enkephalin with potent opiate activity from procine hypothalamus. Biochem Biophys Res Comm 86:153–160.
56. Minamino N, Kangawa K, Chino N, Sakakibara S, Matsuo H. 1981. β-neo-endorphin, a new hypothalmic "big" leu-enkephalin of porcine origin: Its purification and the complete amino acid sequence. Biochem Biophys Res Comm 99:864–870.
57. Minamino N, Kangawa K, Fukuda A, Matsuo H, Iagarashi M. 1980. A new octapeptide related to dynorphin from porcine hypothalamus. Biochem Biophys Res Comm 95:1475–1481.
58. Goldstein A, Fischli W. Lowney LI, Hunkapiller M, Hood L. 1981. Porcine pituitary dynorphin: Complete amino acid sequence of the biologically active heptadecapeptide. Proc Natl Acad Sci USA 78:7219–7223.
59. Fishchli W, Goldstein A, Hunkapiller MW, Hood LE. 1982. Isolation and amino acid sequence analysis of a 4000 Dalton dynorphin from porcine pituitary. Proc Natl Acad Sci USA 79:5435–5437.
60. Kilpatrick DL, Wahlström A, Lahm, HW, Blacher R, Ezra E, Fleminger G, Udenfriend S. 1982. Characterisation of Rimorphin, a new [Leu]enkephalin containing peptide from bovine posterior pituitary glands. Life Sci 31:1849–1852.
61. Kilpatrick DL, Wahlström A, Lahm HW, Blacher R, Udenfriend S. 1982. Rimorphin, a unique, naturally occurring [Leu]enkephalin-containing peptide found in association with dynorphin and α-neo-endorphin. Proc Natl Acad Sci USA 79:6480–6483.
62. Suda M, Nakao K, Yashimasa T, Ikeda Y, Sakamoto M, Yanaihara N, Numa S, Imura H. 1983. A novel opioid peptidc, leumorphin, acts as an agonist at the ϰ opiate receptor. Life Sci 32:2769–2775.
63. Takagi H, Shiomi H, Ueda H, Amano H. 1979. Morphine-like analgesia by a new dipeptide L-tyrosyl-L-arginine (Kyotorphin) and its analogue. Eur J Pharmacol 55:109–111.
64. Takagi H, Shiomi H, Ueda H, Amano H. 1979. A novel analgesic dipeptide from bovine brain is a possible met-enkephalin releaser, Nature (Lond) 282:410–413.
65. Montecucchi PC, De Castiglione R, Piani S, Gozzini L, Erspamer V. 1981. Amino acid composition and sequence of dermorphin, a novel opiate-like peptide from the skin of phyllomedusa sauvages. Int J Peptide Prot Res 17:275–283.
66. Erspamer V, Melchiorri P. 1980. Amphibian skin peptides and mammalian neuropeptides. In Pecile A, Miller EE (eds): Growth Hormone and Other Biologically Active Peptides. Amsterdam: Excerpta Medica, pp. 185–200.
67. Sarne Y, Gothilf Y, Weissman BA. 1980. Humoral endorphin: Endogenous opiate in blood, cerebrospinal fluid and brain. In Way EL (ed): Endogenous and Exogenous Opiate Agonists and Antagonists. Oxford: Pergamon, pp. 317–320.
68. Pert CB, Pert A, Tallman JF. 1976. Isolation of a novel endogenous opiate analgesic from human blood. Proc Natl Acad Sci USA 73:2226–2230.
69. Brantl V, Gramsch C, Lottspeich F, Mertz R Jaeger K-H, Herz A. 1985. Novel opioid peptides derived from mitochondrial cytochrome b: Cytochrophins. Eur J Pharmacol 111: 293–294.
70. Brantl V, Gramsch C, Lottspeich F, Mertz R, Jaeger K-H, Herz A. 1986. Novel opioid peptides derived from hemoglobin: Hemorphins. Eur J Pharmacol 125:309–310.
71. Zioudrou C, Klee WA. 1978. Exorphins — Peptides with opioid activity derived from α-casein and wheat gluten. In van Ree JM, Terenius L (eds): Characteristics and Functions of Opioids. Amsterdam: Elsevier/North Holland Biomedical Press, pp. 243–244.
72. Henschen A, Lottspeich F, Brantl V, Teschemacher H. 1979. Novel opioid peptides derived from casein (β-casomorphins) II. Hoppe-Seyler's. Z Physiol Chem 360:1271–1224.
73. Henschen A, Brantl V, Teschemacher H, Lottspeich F. 1980. β-Casomorphins — novel opioid peptides derived from bovine casein — isolation and structure. In Way EL (ed):

Endogenous and Exogenous Opiate Agonists and Antagonists. Oxford: Pergamon, pp. 233–236.
74. Brantl V. 1984. Novel opioid peptides derived from human β-casein: Human β-casomorphins. Eur J Pharmacol 106:213–214.
75. Meisel H. 1986. Chemical characterization and opioid activity of an exorphin isolated from in vivo digests of casein. FEBS Lett 196:223–227.
76. Chang KJ, Killian A, Hazum E, Cuatrecasas P, Chang JK. 1981. Morphiceptin (NH_4-Tyr-Pro-Phe-Pro-$CONH_2$): A potent and specific agonist for morphine (μ) receptors. Science 212:75–77.
77. Martin WR, Eades CG. Thompson JA, Huppler RE, Gilbert PE, 1976. The effects of morphine- and nalorphine-like drugs in the nondependent and morphine-dependent chronic spinal dog. J Pharmacol Exp Ther 197:517–532.
78. Volozin BL, Pasternak GW. 1981. Classification of multiple morphine and enkephalin binding sites in the central nervous system. Proc Natl Acad Sci USA 78:6181–6185.
79. Lord JAH, Waterfield AA, Hughes J, Kosterlitz HW. 1976. Multiple opiate receptors. In Kosterlitz HW (ed): Opiates and Endogenous Opioid Peptides. Amsterdam: Elsevier/North Holland Biomedical Press, pp. 275–280.
80. Audiger Y, Attali A, Muzarguil H, Cros J. 1982. Characterization of ^3H etorphine binding in guinea pig striatum after blockade of mu and delta sites. Life Sci 31:1287–1290.
81. Attali A, Gouardères C, Mazarguil H, Audiger Y, Cros J. 1982. Differential interaction of opiates of multiple "kappa" binding sites in the guinea-pig lumbo-sacral spinal cord. Life Sci 31:1371–1375.
83. Wüster M, Schultz R, Herz A. 1979. Specificity of opioids towards the μ-, δ- and ε-opiate receptors. Neurosci Lett 15:193–198.
83. Grevel J, Sadee W. 1983. An opiate binding site in the rat brain is highly selective for 4,5-epotymorphinans. Science 221:1198–1200.
84. Smyth DG. 1983. β-Endorphin and related peptides in pituitary, brain, pancreas and antrum. Br Med Bull 39:25–30.
85. Kosterlitz HW. 1985. Opioid peptides and their receptors. Proc R Soc Lond [Biol] 225: 27–40.
86. Zamir N, Palkovits M, Brownstein M. 1985. Distributive of immunoreactive Met-enkephalin Arg 6-Gly 7-Leu 8 and Leu-enkephalin in discrete regions of the rat brain. Brain Res 326:1–8.
87. Zamir N, Weber E. Palkovits M, Brownstein MJ. 1985. Distribution of immunoreactive metorphamide (adrenorphin) in discrete regions of the rat brain: Comparison with Met-enkephalin-Arg 6-Gly 7-Leu 8. Brain Res 361:193–199.
88. Hughes J. 1983. Biogenesis, release and inactivation of enkephalins and dynorphins. Br Med Bull 39:17–24.
89. Martinez J, Potier P. 1986. Peptide hormones as prohormones. TIPS 7:139–147.
90. Weber E, Evans CJ, Barchas JD. 1983. Multiple endogenous ligands for opioid recetprs. TIPS 4:333–336.
91. Smyth DG, Zakarian S. 1981. Selective processing of beta-endorphin in regions of porcine pituitary. Nature 288:613–615.
92. Alassi N, Taylor L, Akil H. 1982. Peptide F (pro-enkephalin fragment): Radioimmunoassay, and stress-induced changes in adrenal. Life Sci 31:1875–1878.
93. Udenfriend S. Kilpatrick DL. 1983. Biochemistry of the enkephalins and enkephalin-containing peptides. Arch Biochem Biophys 221:309–323.
94. Ikada Y, Nakao K, Yoshimasa T, Yanaihara N, Numa S, Imura H. 1982. Existence of met-enkephalin-Arg 6-Gly 7-Leu 8 with Met-enkephalin, Leu-enkephalin and Met-enkephalin-Arg 6-Phe 7 in the brain of guineapig, rat and golden hamster. Biochem Biophys Res Comm 107:656–662.
95. Takagi H, Shiomi H, Fukui K, Hayashi K, Kiso Y, Kitagawa K. 1982. Isolation of a novel analgesic pentapeptide, neokyotorphin from bovine brain. Life Sci 31:1733–1736.
96. Beaumont A. 1983. Putative peptide neurotransmitters: The opioid peptides. Int Rev Exp Pathol 25:279–305.
97. Cuello AC. 1983. Central distribution of opioid peptides. Br Med Bull 39:11–16.
98. Weber E, Roth KA, Barchas JD. 1982. Immunohistochemical distribution of neoendorphin/

dynorphin neuronal systems in rat brain: Evidence for co-localization. Proc Natl Acad Sci USA 79:3062–3066.

99. Frederickson RCA, Geary LE. 1982. Endogenous opioid peptides: Review of physiological, pharmacological and clinical aspects. Prog Neurobiol 19:19–69.
100. Loh HH, Smith AP, Lee NM. 1983. Dynorphin: Pharmacology and clinical implications. In Lemberger L, Riedenberg MM (eds): Proceedings of the Second World Conference on Clinical Pharmacoloy and Therapeutics. Am Soc Pharmacol Exp Ther, pp. 727–732.
101. Frederickson RCA. 1984. Endogenous opioids and related derivatives. In Kuhar M, Pasternak G (eds): Analgesics: Neurochemical, Behavioral, and Clinical Perspectives. New York: Raven Press, pp. 9–68.
102. Fratta W, Yang H-Y, Majane B, Costa E. 1979. Distribution of β-endorphin and related peptides in the hypothalamus and pituitary. Neuroscience 4:1903–1908.
103. Rossier J, Vargo TM, Minick S, Ling N, Bloom FE, Guillemin R. 1977. Regional dissociation of β-endorphin and enkephalin contents in rat brain and pituitary. Proc Natl Acad Sci USA 74:5162–5165.
104. Zakarian S, Smyth D. 1979. Distribution of active and inactive forms of endorphins in rat pituitary and brain. Proc Natl Acad Sci USA 76:5972–5976.
105. Smyth DG, Massey DE, Zakarian S, Finnie MDA. 1979. Endorphins are stored in biologically active and inactive forms: Isolation of α-N-acetyl peptides. Nature 279:252–254.
106. Bloom FE, Battenberg E, Rossier J, Ling N, Guillemin R. 1978. Neurons containing β-endorphin in rat brain exist separately from those containing enkephalin: Immunocytochemical studies. Proc Natl Acad Sci USA 75:1591–1595.
107. Lindberg I, Symthe SJ, Dahl JL. 1979. Regional distribution of enkephalin in bovine brain. Brain Res 168:200–204.
108. Larsson L-I, Childers S, Snyder SH. 1979. Met- and Leu-enkephalin immunoreactivity in separate neurons. Nature 282:407–410.
109. Herz A, Höllt V, Gramsch CH, Seizinger BR. 1982. Differential distribution, release, and modulation of dynorphin and beta-endorphin. Adv Biochem Psychopharmacol 31:51–59.
110. Zamir N, Weber E, Palkovits M, Brownstein M. 1984. Differential processing of prodynorphin and proenkephalin in specific regions of the rat brain. Proc Natl Acad Sci USA 81:6886–6889.
111. Zamir N, Quirion R. 1985. Dynorphinergic pathways of Leu-enkephalin production in the rat brain. Neuropeptides 5:441–444.
112. Zamir N, Palkovits M, Brownstein MJ. 1983. Distribution of immunoreactive dynorphin in the central nervous system of the rat. Brain Res 280:81–93.
113. Zamir N, Palkovits M, Brownstein MJ. 1984. Distribution of immunoreactive dynorphin A (1–8) in discrete nuclei of the rat brain: Comparison with dynorphin A. Brain Res 307: 61–68.
114. Zamir N, Palkovits M, Brownstein MJ. 1984. The distribution of immunoreactive α-neo-endorphin in the central nervous system of the rat. J Neuroscience 4:1248–1252.
115. Zamir N, Palkovits M, Weber E, Brownstein MJ. 1984. Distribution of immunoreactive dynorphin B in discrete areas of the rat brain and spinal cord. Brain Res 300:121–127.
116. Maysinger D, Höllt V, Seizinger BR, Mehracin P, Pasi A, Herz A. 1982. Parallel distribution of immunoreactive α-neo-endorphin and dynorphin in rat and human tissue. Neuropeptides 2:211–225.
117. Palkovits M, Brownstein MJ, Zamir N. 1984. On the origin of dynorphin A and α-neo-endorphin in the substantia nigra. Neuropeptides 4:193–199.
118. Basbaum AI, Fields HL. 1978. Endogenous pain control mechanisms. Review and hypothesis. Ann Neurol 4:451–462.
119. Basbaum AI, Fields HL. 1984. Endogenous pain control systems: Brainstem spinal pathways and endorphin circuitry. Am Rev Neurosci 7:309–338.
120. Melzack R, Wall PD. 1965. Pain mechanism: A new theory. Science 150:971–979.
121. Basbaum AI. 1984. Endorphins and the control of pain: Anatomical studies of enkephalin and dynorphin. In Patou W, Mitchell J, Turner P (eds): Proceedings of IUPHAR 9th International Congress of Pharmacology, Vol.1 London: pp. 359–365.
122. Khachaturian H, Watson SJ, Lewis ME, Coy D, Goldstein A, Akil H. 1982. Dynorphin immunocytochemistry in the rat central nervous sytem. Peptides 3:941–954.
123. Bloom FE, Battenberg E, Rossier J, Ling N, Guillemin R. 1978. Neurons containing β-

endorphin in rat brain exist separately from those containing enkephalin: Immunocytochemical studies. Proc Natl Acad Sci USA 75:1591–1595.
124. Höllt V, Tulunay C, Woo SK, Loh H, Herz A. 1982. Opioid peptides derived from proenkephalin A but not from pro-enkephalin B are substantial analgesics after administration into brain of mice. Eur J Pharmacol 83:355–356.
125. Tulunay FC, Jen MF, Change JK, Loh HH, Lee NM. 1981. Possible regulatory role of dynorphin on morphine and β-endorphin-induced analgesia. J Pharmacol Exp Ther 219: 296–298.
126. Elde R, Hökfelt T, Johansson O, Terenius L. 1976. Immunohistochemical studies using antibodies to leucine-enkephalin: Initial observations on the nervous system of the rat. Neuroscience 1:349–351.
127. Glazer EJ, Basbaum AI. 1981. Immunohistochemical localization of leucine-enkephalin in the spinal cord of the cat. Enkephalin-containing marginal neurons and pain modulation. J Comp Neurol 196:377–389.
128. Glazer EJ, Basbaum AI. 1983. Opioid neurons and pain modulation: An ultrastructural analysis of enkephalin in cat superficial dorsal horn. Neuroscience 10:357–376.
129. Vincent SR, Hökfelt T, Christensson I, Terenius L. 1982. Dynorphin-immunoreactive neurons in the central nervous system of the rat. Neurosci Lett 33:185–190.
130. Barnard EA, Demoliou-Mason C. 1983. Molecular properties of opioid receptors. Br Med Bull 39:37–45.
131. Huidebro-Toro JP, Way EL. 1985. Opiates. In Grahame-Smith DG (ed): Psychopharmacology 2, Part 1: Preclinical Psychopharmacology. Amsterdam: Elsevier Science Publishers, pp. 283–342.
132. Law PY, Harris RA, Loh HH, Way EL. 1978. Evidence for the involvement of cerebroside sulfatein opiate receptor binding. Studies with Azure A and Jimpy mutant mice. J Pharmacol Exp Ther 207:458–468.
133. Craves FB, Zale B, Leybin L, Baumann N, Loh HH. 1980. Antibodies to cerebroside sulfate inhibit the effects of morphine and β-endorphin. Science 207:75–76.
134. Zukin RS, Zukin SR. 1984. The case for multiple opiate receptors. TINS 7:160–164.
135. Wood PL. 1982. Multiple opiate receptors: Support for unique mu, delta and kappa sites. Neuropharmacology 21:487–497.
136. Paterson SJ, Robson LE, Kosterlitz HW. 1984. Opioid receptors. In Udenfriend S, Meienhofer J (eds): The Peptides, Analysis, Synthesis and Biology, Vol. 6. New York: Academic Press, pp. 147–189.
137. Kosterlitz HW, Paterson SJ. 1985. Types of opioid receptors: Relation to antinociception. Philos Trans R Soc Lond [Biol] 308:291–297.
138. Pleuvry BJ. 1983. An update on opioid receptors. Br J Anaesth 55:143S–146S.
139. Pasternak GW. 1986. Biochemistry and pharmacology of multiple mu opioid receptors. In Foley KM, Inturissi CE (eds): Advances in Pain Research and Therapy. Vol. 8. New York: Raven Press, pp. 337–350.
140. Schulz R, Wuster M, Kreuss H, Herz A. 1980. Selective development of tolerance without dependence in multiple opiate receptors of mouse vas deferens. Nature 285:242–243.
141. North RA. 1986. Opioid receptor types and membrane ion channels. TIPS 7:114–155.
142. Oka T, Negishi K, Suda M, Matsuniya T, Inazu T. Ueki M. 1981. Rabbit vas deferens. A specific bioassay for opioid κ-receptor agonists. Eur J Pharmacol 73:235–236.
143. Schulz R, Wuster M, Rubini P, Herz A. 1981. Functional opiate receptors in the guinea-pig ileum: Their differentations by means of selective tolerance development. J Pharmacol Exp Ther 219:547–550.
144. Chavkin C, Goldstein A. 1981. Specific receptor for the opioid peptide dynorphin: Structure–activity relationships. Proc Natl Acad Sci USA 78:6543–6547.
145. James IF, Chavkin C, Goldstein C. 1982. Selectivity of dynorphin for K opioid receptors. Life Sci 31:1331–1334.
146. Schulz R, Wüster M, Herz A. 1981. Pharmacological characterization of the ε-opiate receptor. J Pharmacol Exp Ther 216:604–606.
147. Zukin S. 1982. Differing stereospecificities distinguish opiate receptor subtypes. Life Sci 31:1307–1310.
148. Pert CB, Kuhar MJ, Snyder SH. 1976. Opiate receptor: Autoradiographic localization in rat brain. Proc Natl Acad Sci USA 73:3729–3733.

149. Foote RW, Maurer R. 1982. Autoradiographic localization of opiate κ-receptors in the guinea-pig brain. Eur J Pharmacol 85:99–103.
150. Lewis ME, Khachaturian H, Watson SJ. 1982. Visualization of opiate receptors and opioid peptides in sequential brain sections. Life Sci 31:1347–1350.
151. Quirion R, Zajac JM, Morgat JL, Roque BP. 1983. Autoradiographic distribution of mu and delta opiate receptors in rate brain using highly selective ligands. Life Sci 33 (Suppl I): 227–230.
152. Wamsley JK. 1983. Opioid receptors: Autoradiography. Pharmacol Rev 35:69–83.
153. Goodman RR, Snyder SH. 1982 Kappa opiate receptors localized by autoradiography to deep layers of cerebral cortex: Relation to sedative effects. Proc Natl Acad Sci USA 79: 5703–5707.
154. Chang K-J, Cooper BR, Hazum E, Cuatrecases P. 1979. Multiple opiate receptors: Different regional distribution in the brain and differential binding of opiates and opioid peptides. Mol Pharmacol 16:91–104.
155. Zukin SR, Fitz-Syage ML, Nichtenhauser R, Zukin RS. 1983. Specific binding of [^{3}H] phenylcyclidine in rat central nervous tissue: Further characterization and technical considerations. Brain Res 258:277–284.
156. Robson LE, Paterson SJ, Kosterlitz HW. 1983. Opiate Receptors. In Iversen L, Iversen SD, Snyder SH (eds): Handbook of Psychopharmacology. New York: Plenum Press, pp. 13–80.
157. Quirion R, Hammer R, Herkenham M, Pert CB. 1981. Phenyl-cyclidine (angel dust)/sigma "opiate" recetors. Visualization by tritium-sensitive film. Proc Natl Acad Sci USA 78: 5881–5885.
158. Goodman RR, Snyder SH, Kuhar MJ, Young WS III. 1980. Differentiation of delta and mu opiate recetor localizations by light microscopic autoradiography. Proc Natl Acad Sci USA 77:6239–6243.
159. Goodman RR, Snyder SH. 1982. Autoradiographic localization of kappa opiate receptors to deep layers of the cerebral cortex may explain unique sedative and analgesic effects. Life Sci 21:1291–1294.
160. Duka TH, Schubert P, Wuster M, Stoiber R, Herz A. 1981. A selective distribution pattern of different opiate receptors in certain areas of rat brain as revealed by in vitro autoradiography. Neurosci Lett 21:119–124.
161. Yaksh TL, Yeung JC, Rudy TA. 1976. Systematic examination in the rat of brain sites sensitive to the direct application of morphine: Observation of differential effects within the periaqueductal gray. Brain Res 114:83–103.
162. Yaksh TL, Rudy TA. 1978. Narcotic analgesics: CNS sites and mechanisms of action as revealed by intracerebral injection techniques. Pain 4:299–359.
163. Bennett GJ, Mayer PJ. 1979. Inhibition of spinal cord interneurons by narcotic microinjection and focal electrical stimulation in the periaqueductal central gray matter. Brain Res 172:243–257.
164. Pert CB, Pert A. Chang JK, Fond BTW. 1976. [D-Ala^2]-Met-enkephalinamide: A potent, long-lasting synthetic pentapeptide analgesic. Science 194:330–332.
165. Jacquet YF. 1978. Opiate effects after adrenocorticotropin or β-endorphin injection in the periaqueductal gray matter of rats. Science 201:1032–1034.
166. Wood PL, Rackham A, Richard J. 1981. Spinal analgesia: Comparison of the mu agonist morphine and the kappa agonist ethylketazocine. Life Sci 28:2119–2125.
167. Nordberg G. 1984. Pharmacokinetic aspects of spinal morphine analgesia. Acta Anesthesiol Scand 28 (Suppl 79): 1–38.
168. Onofrio BM, Yaksh TL. 1983. Intrathecal delta-receptor ligand produces analgesia in man. Lancet i:1386–1387.
169. Coombs DW, Saunders RL. Lachance D, Savage S, Ragnarsson TS, Jensen LE. 1985. Intrathecal morphine tolerance: Use of intrathecal clonidine, DADLE and intraventricular morphine. Anesthesiology 62:358–363.
170. Tung AS, Yaksh TL. 1982. *In vivo* evidence for multiple opiate receptors mediating analgesia in the rat spinal cord. Brain Res 247:75–83.
171. Han JS, Xie CW. 1982. Dynorphin: Potent analgesic effect in the spinal cord of the rat. Life Sci 31:1781–1784.
172. Piercey MF, Lahti RA, Schroeder LA, Einspahr FJ, Barsuhn C. 1982. U 50488H, a pure kappa receptor agonist with spinal analgesic loci in the mouse. Life Sci 31:1197–1200.

173. Morley JS. 1983. Chemistry of opioid peptides. Br Med Bull 39:5–10.
174. Takemori AE, Ikeda M, Portoghese PS. 1986. The μ, κ and δ properties of various opioid agonists. Eur J Pharmacol 123:357–361.
175. Nordberg G, Hedner T. 1988. Spinal opiates — pharmacokinetic aspects. In Löfström B, Sjöstrand U (eds): Local Anaesthesia and Regional Blockade. Amsterdam: Elsevier Science Publishers B.V, pp. 221–243.

2. SYSTEMIC AND LOCAL DISTRIBUTION OF OPIOIDS AFTER SPINAL ADMINISTRATION: IMPLICATIONS FOR THEIR CLINICAL USE

LARS L. GUSTAFSSON

Spinal opioid analgesia may be achieved either by epidural or intrathecal administration. The analgesic effect is exerted through the binding of drugs to opioid receptors in the dorsal horn of the spinal cord [1, 2]. The fraction of the dose that reaches the intended site of action in the spinal cord is lower with epidural than with intrathecal administration because of the high blood flow and pronounced distribution into the systemic circulation in the first case. Similar therapeutic and toxic effects can be present irrespective of the route of administration when equipotent doses are given.

Spinal opioid analgesia is of clinical benefit only if its efficacy is greater, and the incidence of side effects acceptable, when compared with administration by other routes. Few such comparisons have been performed, especially in the treatment of patients with cancer pain [3]. Several opioids (e.g., buprenorphine, diamorphine, fentanyl, hydromorphone, morphine, methadone, pentazocine, and pethidine) have been applied by the spinal route to test their efficacy in various pain conditions in humans [4]. Recently, epidural alfentanil [5] and lofentanil [6] were reported to achieve long-lasting analgesia with few side effects. Published results conflict, so the advantages and disadvantages of different opioids in achieving spinal opioid analgesia remain unclear. Epidural administration of morphine to control postoperative pain is, however, based on results from a number of well-designed clinical studies [4].

This chapter discusses general aspects of systemic and local distribution of opioids applied by the spinal route. Pharmacokinetic results important to the selection of appropriate opioids for the clinical setting will be evaluated. Results from studies on drug disposition in various species will be reviewed in relation to their relevance to drug administration in humans.

FACTORS AFFECTING EFFICACY OF OPIOIDS APPLIED ON THE SPINAL ROUTE

The onset and duration of spinal opioid analgesia are determined by the pharmacokinetics, receptor affinity, and intrinsic activity of each opioid administered. The characteristics of distribution processes into the spinal cord, into cerebrospinal fluid (CSF), and into the systemic circulation of a specific opioid are more important for the onset of spinal opioid analgesia and the duration of its effect than other pharmacokinetic parameters, such as metabolic pathways and excretory routes. Physiochemical characteristics of the drug affect the rate of diffusion from CSF into the dorsal horn of the spinal cord. Lipophilic opioids show the shortest time to onset of analgesia, both in animals and man [1, 2, 7, 8], whereas hydrophilic drugs induce the longest duration of effect [4, 7, 8] (table 2–1).

ANTINOCICEPTION OF SPINAL OPIOIDS IN ANIMALS: PHARMACODYNAMIC VERSUS PHARMACOKINETIC FACTORS

Dose-dependent antinociceptive effects in experimental models have been demonstrated after intrathecal administration of several μ-agonists such as lofentanil, morphine, sufentanil, fentanyl, alfentanil, methadone, and pethidine in the rat [9, 10]. Partial agonists to μ- and/or K-receptors such as buprenorphine and pentazocine show less impressive effects [11]. For some drugs, dose-dependent antinociceptive effects have also been demonstrated in other species, including primates [12]. Of several drugs tested in equipotent doses, long-lasting analgesia has so far been seen only with the hydrophilic drug morphine and with a single lipophilic drug, lofentanil [10]. The results of epidural administration of opioids in animals are not as clear as with intrathecal administration because of methodological problems discussed below.

Recently it has been found that lipophilic compounds (alfentanil, sufentanil, and lofentanil) can produce similar analgesic effects in animals whether the same dose is given by the epidural or by the intravenous route [13, 14]. Morphine, a hydrophilic compound, was much more potent after epidural administration than after intravenous administration [13]. These results can be explained by the fact that lipophilic opioids bind to spinal cord opioid receptors to the same extent whether the drug is given by intravenous or by epidural route [14]. It is unlikely that these results were affected by methodological problems encountered after chronic catherization of the epidural space in animals.

Results from experimental studies should be interpreted critically, since methodological problems may affect the distribution of the drug, especially after epidural administration [12, 13]. Within a few weeks, fibrosis may de-

Table 2–1. Analgesic effects versus lipophilicity. Opioids administered by the epidural route in approximately equipotent doses (maximal effect) in humans

Drug	Partition coefficient[1]	Dose (mg)	Onset[2] (min)	Duration[3] (hours)	Type of postoperative pain	Reference
Morphine	1.4	4–4.5	60–120	14–16	Knee arthrotomy	30
		6–7	36 ± 6	19.5 ± 5.0	Lower abdominal	31
Hydromorphone	1–2 (?)	1.2–1.3	22.5 ± 6	9.8 ± 5.5	Abdominal	31
Pethidine	38.8	60	15	1–2	Hip replacement	36
		60	?	6.6 ± 3.3	Various	37
Methadone	116	8.8	10–20	5.6 ± 2.7	Abdominal	31
Alfentanil	129	1.8–2	5	0.8–1	Various	5
Fentanyl	813	0.1	10–20	2–3	Various	38
Lofentanil	1450	0.005	<10	12–20	Lower extremity	6

[1] Octanol/pH 7.4 buffer partition coefficient. A hydrophilic compound has a low and a lipophilic drug a high value.
[2] Usually the time until full effect.
[3] Mean values.

velop around an epidural catheter in rats and probably in primates [12, 13]. In rats, after ten days of implantation the analgesic effect of epidural morphine was only 20%–25% of the initial results [13]. With the more lipophilic drugs fentanyl and alfentanil, the corresponding figures were 35%–50% [13].

The analgesic potency of intrathecal morphine was substantially higher than intrathecal meperidine (pethidine) in primates with chronically implanted catheters, whereas epidural morphine and meperidine showed the same low potency [12]. Fibrotic processes around the epidural catheter notably affect the analgesic effect most for slowly diffusing hydrophilic drugs. The diminishing analgesic effect sometimes observed in man may be explained by low CSF concentrations of morphine secondary to impaired diffusion because of fibrosis around epidural catheters implanted for chronic use [15].

PHARMACOKINETICS OF SPINAL OPIOIDS IN ANIMALS

The disposition of spinal opioids in different species is not well characterized. In dogs, around 50% (range 6% to 100%) of the epidural dose of morphine was recovered in the azygous vein during the initial hour after injection [16]. Less than 1% of the dose was calculated to cross the dura mater in an experiment involving only a few dogs [16]. Deposition in epidural fat tissue may be a significant route to initial transfer besides systemic uptake for lipophilic drugs [17].

Systematic studies on the various distribution routes of opioids within the central nervous system have been performed only after intraventricular drug administration [18]. Within five minutes of intraventricular application, lipophilic compounds such as etorphine and fenanyl were rapidly transported into the systemic circulation (50% of the dose), whereas hydrophilic agents including hydromorphone and morphine showed a low rate of transfer (3%–5%) [18]. The relative potency of intraventricular versus intravenous administration correlated inversely to lipophilicity in 11 tested opioids [18].

The fraction of the intrathecal or epidural dose that distributes into the spinal cord will, in a similar way, correlate to the lipophilicity of the drug. Only 7% of an intrathecal dose of meperidine, but as much as 27% of morphine, was recovered in the spinal cord of the rat at 15 minutes after injection [19]. These results accord with the short-lived effect of meperidine and long-lasting analgesia after morphine administration [8]. However, lofentanil shows long-lasting analgesia despite its lipophilicity and its rapid distribution from the spinal cord [13]. This is because of an extremely pronounced receptor affinity [13].

The amount of an intrathecal or epidural dose that is ultimately transferred rostrally in the cerebrospinal fluid is not known. Distribution by this route is of minor importance for overall disposition, but high doses may induce severe side effects, such as nausea, vomiting, and ventilatory depression, since appreciable amounts of the drug will diffuse into supraspinal control centers such as the brainstem respiratory center. Meperidine showed a relatively lower tendency to spread rostrally than morphine, both in rats undergoing intrathecal administration and in monkeys received intrathecal or epidural drug

[19, 20]. Temporally, appearance of maximal drug concentrations in the cisterna magna was independent of the particular opioid administered, indicating that CSF bulk flow determines the time delay between injection and arrival appearance of drugs in rostral parts of the CSF system [4].

PHARMACOKINETICS OF SPINAL OPIOIDS IN HUMANS

Data on disposition of spinal opioids in humans are incomplete, since medical risks exclude sampling of CSF from rostral levels in most cases. Moreover, there are no reliable noninvasive techniques to quantify distribution processes into the spinal cord. The major routes of distribution of opioids after epidural and intrathecal administration, respectively, are listed in table 2–2.

Drug transfer into the vascular system

Uptake into the vascular system is the major route of distribution of epidural opioids, irrespective of their physiochemical properties. This means that the blood flow of the extradural space is more important than physiochemical properties for the rate of systemic uptake of opioids. In fact, plasma concentrations of morphine after epidural administration are in the same range as when given by intramuscular injection [4, 21]. It has been calculated that at most 1%–2% of the epidural dose is transferred into the CSF [22]. It would therefore be difficult to detect differences in the rate of dural transfer between drugs with various physiochemical properties. However, the rate of distribution into both systemic circulation and into the CSF will be larger for lipophilic than hydrophilic opioids [23].

Less than 4% of the administered dose is present in the CSF or spinal cord, whether meperidine (pethidine) or morphine is given. Greater amounts of morphine than of pethidine are found in the spinal cord, both at lumbar and thoracic levels. These theoretical calculations are based on published CSF concentrations [24] and on experimental studies of opioid concentrations at various levels of the spinal cord in rats [19].

Clinical doses of intrathecal morphine (0.25–0.5 mg) produce almost undetectable plasma concentrations of morphine [25], whereas an intrathecal dose of 14 mg morphine gives only slightly lower plasma concentrations than after epidural administration [26]. However, plasma peak levels occur later after intrathecal (at 30–60 minutes after dose) than after epidural (10–15 minutes) administration [26]. Plasma concentrations of lipophilic drugs would be similar whether the compounds are given by the intrathecal or epidural route, since such drugs diffuse rapidly into vessels draining the spinal cord. In fact, the lipophilic compound meperidine shows the same potency in primates regardless of its route of administration [9].

Drug transfer into the CSF

CSF concentrations of morphine and meperidine (limited data) have been assayed after spinal drug administration [4, 21, 25, 27]. Near the site of injection, CSF concentration of morphine are 100–200 times and 1000–5000 times

Table 2–2. Distribution routes of spinal opioids in humans

	Epidural route	Intrathecal route
Distribution into the systemic circulation	a. Uptake into blood vessels of the epidural space b. Uptake into vessels draining the spinal cord	Uptake into vessels draining the spinal cord. Improtant route.
Spread within the epidural space	Minor route unless a large volume is injected	No
Deposition in fat tissue of the extradural space	May be of importance for lipophilic opioids	No
Paravertebral elimination	Possible	Not relevant
Passage over the dura	A minor part of the dose. Less than 1%–2% of an epidural dose of morphine [21]	Not relevant
Transfer within CSF	Part of the dose in CSF may be transported in rostral or caudal direction Maximal morphine concentrations of CSF at cervical level may be expected 3–6 hours after lumbar administration [4]	As for extradural dose administration. Increased risks for rostral transfer when large volumes are used
Spinal cord	A minor part of the dose reaches the site of action	A major part of the dose diffuses into the spinal cord. Systemic uptake is through the vessels draining the spinal cord

higher than in plasma after epidural and intrathecal administration, respectively [21, 25]. Up to nine-fold interindividual differences in lumbar CSF concentrations of morphine have been observed with a weight-adjusted dose of the drug [28]. These variations in CSF concentrations may partly explain the differences in duration of analgesia observed clinically [4]. A few hours after administration, the elimination half-life of morphine in CSF is similar to that calculated from plasma data (around 3–4 hours), since elimination from CSF should be in equilibrium with drug elimination from plasma.

Some pharmacokinetic differences between intrathecal and epidural drug administration may be relevant to the mechanism of action. After intrathecal administration of morphine, supraspinal influences on the analgesic effect through systemic absorption seem unlikely, since negligible plasma concentrations of morphine are detected. In contrast, supraspinal factors may well influence the effect of epidural morphine, since systemic uptake yields similar plasma concentrations to those following intramuscular administration. There is also experimental evidence that simultaneous injections of morphine at spinal and supraspinal levels achieve a magnitude of analgesia that to duplicate would require greater spinal doses. [29]

Spinal cord distribution

Most of an intrathecal dose reaches the vascular system after diffusion into vessels draining the spinal cord, whereas at most a few percent of an epidural dose is distributed into the system circulation by this route. No human data exist on how physiochemical properties of opioids affect the rate of diffusion into the spinal cord. Since analgesic effects of various opioids in man agree with experimental results in animals, the data on distribution of opioids in animals theoretically would be valid in humans also.

Maximal analgesic effect occurs no earlier than at 60 minutes and at 30–40 minutes after administration of morphine by the epidural and intrathecal route, respectively [30, 31, 32]. This implies that diffusion into the spinal cord rather than dural transfer would be rate-limiting for onset of analgesia after extradural administration of hydrophilic drug.

These results are in accord with the slower onset of effect of hydrophilic drugs after epidural compared to after intrathecal administration. Confirmation of this issue in man awaits the results from comparisons of the two routes of administration in the same individuals; such comparisons should determine whether clinically important differences to onset of analgesia exist.

Rostral transport within CSF

After subarachnoid injection of a drug, rostral transport may occur by CSF bulk flow or by unknown mechanisms within the neuraxis (table 2–2). A drug that is injected into the epidural space may reach supraspinal centers by these two routes and be spread within the extradural space itself. Transport by CSF bulk flow seems to be the route of quantitative importance.

The distribution of drugs from the site of injection after spinal application cannot be compared to the kinetics of radioactively labeled compounds (e.g., ^{131}I-albumin, ^{99}Tc-albumin or radio-iodinated antifibrinogen) [4], since these compounds have molecular weights of 67,000 and 340,000 compared to only 250 to 350 for most drugs. These large molecules have slow diffusion rates through membranes, so a greater fraction of the injected dose reaches supra-spinal regions by CSF bulk flow instead of by being taken up systemically. The rostral spread of an intrathecal dose may be influenced by the administered volume, since a direct relation exists between the volume injected intrathecally and its rostral spread in primates [32]. A large volume increases the CSF pressure rapidly such that rostral transport occurs. Therefore, peak drug concentrations of cisternal CSF occur early after drug administration (at 15–30 minutes) in contrast to delayed peak levels when the drug is transported by CSF bulk flow.

There are few human studies in which concentrations of various opioids in the CSF have been assayed simultaneously at lumbar and cervical levels after epidural drug administration. Lipophilic drugs should be detected in low and hydrophilic compounds in high concentrations in cisternal CSF, since the rate of diffusion into the spinal cord is directly related to the lipophilicity of the drug. In fact, methadone (lipophilic) and morphine (hydrophilic) were detected in low and high concentrations, respectively, at cisternal CSF in a few patents [3].

Adverse effects such as ventilatory depression and vomiting may occur 4–6 hours after spinal administration of morphine at the lumbar level [33, 34, 35]. These symptoms start when significant amounts of the drug have been transported rostrally by CSF bulk flow and have reached vital control centers by diffusion into the floor of the fourth ventricle and medulla. Peak levels of cisternal morphine concentrations precede maximal ventilatory depression because of slow diffusion of morphine into the brain tissue. The incidence and severity of these adverse effects are dose-dependent [4].

IMPLICATIONS

The potency of morphine applied by the spinal route in higher than after intravenous administration. Morphine induces a long-lasting analgesic effect after spinal administration since distribution of the drug from the spinal cord into the systemic circultation is slow. High morphine concentrations will consequently be prolonged at the opioid receptors. Since lipophilic opioids are rapidly distributed from the spinal cord, short-lived effects are expected unless an extremely high receptor affinity of the drug compensates for this. Lofentanil is the single lipophilic opioid tested that shows long-lasting analgesic effects in animals and man. Its use by the spinal route in doubtful since similar duration of effects have been observed whether the same dose is given by the intravenous or by the epidural route in rats [13].

A regional type of spinal morphine analgesia is achieved only when small doses are administered because the drug otherwise will be transported rostrally in significant amounts by CSF bulk flow. Lipophilic drugs will achieve more regional analgesic effects, but frequent administration will be necessary.

Human studies that conclude that lipophilic μ-agonists provide potent and long-lasting analgesia after spinal administration should be interpreted with caution. Today, pharmacokinetic and/or pharmacodynamic factors support use of single dose administration of such drugs by the spinal route instead of intravenous use.

ACKNOWLEDGEMENTS

This work was supported by grants from the Swedish Medical Research Council (3902, 8951) and the Karolinska Institute. Dr. Tom Perry helped with the linguistic revision of the manuscript. Expert secretarial assistance was provided by Gunhild Larsson and Hjördis Oscarson.

REFERENCES

1. Yaksh TL, Noueihed R. 1985. The physiology and pharmacology of spinal opiates. Ann Rev Pharmacol Toxicol 25:433–462.
2. Yaksh TL. 1981. Spinal opiate analgesia: Characteristics and principles of action. Pain 11: 293–346.
3. Max MB, Inturrisi CE, Kaiko RF, Grabinski PY, Li CH, Foley KM. 1985. Epidural and intrathecal opiates: Cerebrospinal fluid and plasma profiles in patients with chronic cancer pain. Clin Pharmacol Ther 38:631–641.
4. Gustafsson LL. 1985. Spinal opiate analgesia: Clinical and experimental aspects. Thesis, Karolinska Institute, Stockholm.
5. Chauvin M, Salbaing J, Perrin D, Levron JC, Viars P. 1985. Clinical assessment and plasma pharmacokinetcs associated with intramuscular or extradural alfentanil. Br J Anaesth 57: 886–891.
6. Bilsbach P, Rolly G, Tampubolon O. 1985. Efficacy of the extradural administration of lofentanil, buprenorphine or saline in the management of postoperative pain. A double-blind study. Br J Anaesth 57:943–948.
7. Cousins MJ, Mather LE. 1984. Intrathecal and epidural administration of opioids. Anesthesiology 61:276–310.
8. Gustafsson LL, Post C. 1986. The degree of analgesia correlates to spinal morphine concentrations after intrathecal administration in rats. Acta Pharmacol Toxicol 58:243–248.
9. Yaksh TL, Rudy TA 1977. Studies on the direct spinal action of narcotics in the production of analgesia in rat. J Pharmacol Ther 202:411–428.
10. Yaksh TL, Noueihed R, Durant PAC. 1986. Studies of the pharmacology and pathology of intrathecally administered 4-anilinopiperidine analogues and morphine in the rat and cat. Anesthesiology 64:54–66.
11. Bryant RM, Olley JE, Tyers MB. 1983. Antinociceptive actions of morphine and buprenorphine given intrathecally in the conscious rat. Br J Pharmacol 78:659–663.
12. Yaksh TL, Reedy SVR. 1981. Studies in the primate on the analgetic effects associated with intrathecal opiates, alfa-adrenergic agonists and baclofen. Anesthesiology 54:451–467.
13. Durant PAC, Yaksh TL. 1986. Epidural injections of bupivacaine, morphine, fentanyl, lofentanil, and DADL in chronically implanted rats: A pharmacologic and pathologic study. Anesthesiology 64:43–53.
14. Colpaert FC, Leysen JE, Michiels M, van den Hoogen RHWM. 1986. Epidural and intravenous sufentanil in the rat: Analgesia, opiate receptor binding, and drug concentrations in plasma and brain. Anesthesiology 65:41–49.
15. Rodan BA, Cohen FL, Bean WJ, Martyack SN. 1985. Fibrous mass complicating epidural morphine infusion. Neurosurgery 16:68–70.
16. Durant PAC, Yaksh TL. 1986. Distribution in cerebrospinal fluid, blood, and lymph of

epidurally injected morphine and insulin in dogs. Anesth Analg 65:583–592.
17. Tucker GT, Mather LE. 1975. Pharmacokinetics of local anaesthetic agents. Br J Anaesth 47:213–224.
18. Herz A, Teschemacher HJ. 1971. Activities and sites of antinociceptive action of morphine-like analgesics and kinetics of distribution following intravenous, intracerebral and intraventricular application. In Herper WJ, Simmonds AB (eds): Advances in Drug Research and Therapy, Vol. 6. New York: Academic Press, pp. 79–119.
19. Gustafsson LL, Post C, Edvardsen B, Ramsay CH. 1985. Distribution of morphine and meperidine after intrathecal administration in rat and mouse. Anesthesiology 63:483–489.
20. Gustafsson LL, Hartvig P, Bergström K, Lundqvist H. Lindberg BS, Långström B, Svärd H, Rane A, Tamsen A. 1989. Distribution of C-labelled morphine and pethidine after spinal administration to Rhesus monkey. Acta Anaesthesiol Scand 33:105–111.
21. Nordberg G, Hedner T, Mellstrand T, Dahlström B. 1983. Pharmacokinetic aspects of epidural morphine analgesia. Anesthesiology 58:545–551.
22. Nordberg G. 1986. Epidural versus intrathecal route of opioid administration. Int Anesthesiol Clin 24:93–111.
23. Watson J, Moore A, McQuay H, Teddy P, Baldwin D, Allen M, Bullingham R. 1984. Plasma morphine concentrations and analgesic effects of lumbar epidural morphine and heroin. Anesth Analg 63:629–634.
24. Tamsen A, Sjöström S, Hartvig P, Persson P, Gabrielsson J, Paalzow L. 1983. CSF and plasma kinetics of morphine and meperidine administration. Anesthesiology 59:A196.
25. Nordberg G, Hedner T, Mellstrand T, Dahlström B. 1984. Pharmacokinetic aspects of intrathecal morphine analgesia. Anesthesiology 60:448–454.
26. Chauvin M, Samii K, Schermann JM, Sandouk P, Bourdon R, Viars P. 1982. Plasma pharmacokinetics of morphine after i.m., extradural, and intrathecal administration. Br J Anaesth 54:843–847.
27. Glynn CJ, Mather LE, Cousins MJ, Graham JR, Wilson PR, 1981. Peridural meperidine in humans: Analgetic response, pharmacokinetics and transmission into CSF. Anesthesiology 55:520–526.
28. Gustafsson LL, Grell AM, Garle M, Rane A, Schildt B. 1984. Kinetics of morphine in cerebrospinal fluid after epidural administration. Acta Anaesthesiol Scand 28:535–539.
29. Yeung JC, Rudy TA. 1980. Multiplicative interactions between narcotic agonisms expressed at spinal and supraspinal sites of antinociceptive action as revealed by concurrent intrathecal and intracerebroventricular injections of morphine. J Pharmacol Exp Ther 215:633–642.
30. Gustafsson LL, Friberg-Nielsen S, Garle M, Mohall A, Rane A, Schildt B, Symreng T. 1982. Epidural and parenteral morphine: Kinetics and effects in postoperative pain in a controlled clinical study. Br J Anaesth 544:1167–1174.
31. Bromage PR, Camporesi E, Chestnut D. 1980. Epidural narcotics for postoperative analgesia. Anesth Analg 59:473–480.
32. Baraka A, Noueihe R, Haij S. 1981. Intrathecal injection of morphine for obstetric analgesia. Anesthesiology 54:136–140.
33. Rawal N, Wattwil M. 1984. Respiratory depression after epidural morphine — an experimental and clinical study. Anesth Analg 63:8–14.
34. Bromage PR, Comporesi EM, Durant PAC, Nielsen CH. 1982. Rostral spread of epidural morphine. Anesthesiology 56:431–436.
35. Bromage PR, Comporesi EM, Durant PAC, Nielsen CH. 1982. Nonrespiratory side effects of epidural morphine. Anesth Analg 61:490–495.
36. Gustafsson LL, Johannisson J, Garle M. 1986. Extradural and parenteral pethidine as analgesia after total hip replacement: Effects and kinetics. A controlled clinical study. Eur J Clin Pharmacol 29:529–534.
37. Torda TA, Pybus DA. 1982. Comparison of four narcotic analgesics for epidural analgesia. Br J Anaesth 54:291–295.
38. Rutter DV, Shewes DG, Morgan M. 1981. Extradural opioids for postoperative analgesia. A double-blind comparison of pethidine, fentanyl and morphine. Br J Anaesth 915–920.

3. INDICATIONS FOR THE USE OF INTRASPINAL OPIOIDS

NARINDER RAWAL

Following identification of highly specific opioid receptors in the brain and spinal cord of animals and man in 1973 [1, 2], it was demonstrated in 1976 that intrathecal morphine produced antinociception in rats [3]. The first clinical use of the technique for the treatment of cancer pain was reported in 1979 [4]. Today, ten years and several hundred international publications later, the technique of injecting opioids epidurally and intrathecally for the management of acute and chronic pain is well established. Although this modality is not the panacea early reports appeared to promise, its place as a major advance in the management of acute and chronic pain is beyond doubt. This chapter will attempt to provide the current indications for the use of epidural and intrathecal opioids.

A recent nationwide follow-up survey in Sweden showed that the administration of epidural opioids has increased greatly during the past five years. Nearly all anesthesia departments used the technique, and epidural opioid analgesia constituted about 25% of all epidural blocks performed in the country [5]. The major indications for the technique were the management of perioperative and postoperative pain, traumatic pain, and chronic malignant pain (figure 3–1). Similar findings were reported in a 1984 review article [6].

The segmental analgesia produced by injecting small amounts of opioids near receptor sites has a role in the treatment of many painful disorders. Thus, in addition to the management of pain associated with surgery, trauma, labor, and cancer, epidural and intrathecal opioids have been successfully used in the

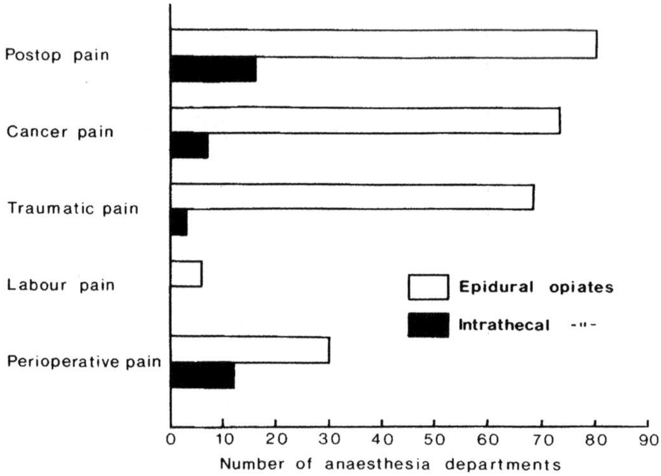

Figure 3–1. Indications for the use of epidural and intrathecal opioids in Sweden. Figure shows the number of anesthesia departments using the technique. Data are from a nationwide follow-up survey in 1985. Total number of anesthesia departments in Sweden is 93.
Source: [5]. (Reproduced with permission.)

treatment of such nonsurgical painful conditions as myocardial infarction, nephrolithiasis, herpes zoster, and thrombophlebitis. Encouraging results have also been reported in the treatment of chronic nonmalignant conditions such as causalgia, low back pain, and ischemic pain. Also, spasticity of spinal or cerebral origin has been managed by epidural and intrathecal administration of opioids, as well as by nonopioids such as midazolam and baclofen [6, 7, 8]. However, there are some areas where epidural and intrathecal opioids are less promising. The doses of morphine that provide excellent postoperative pain relief are inadequate for labor pain. Larger doses of morphine or lipophilic opioids such as fentanyl are more effective, but the results have generally been disappointing. Chapters 1 and 2 cover this aspect of spinal opioid analgesia at length. Also, the perioperative and postoperative stress response is not completely eliminated by epidural or intrathecal opioids (Chapter 4). Furthermore, the technique is associated with distressing or potentially dangerous complications; these are discussed in chapter 5.

POSTOPERATIVE PAIN

There appears to be an awakening of interest in the management of postoperative pain as evidenced by the availability of newer analgesics and by several recent studies of agonist and agonist/antagonist opioids and also their administration via novel routes such as transdermal [9], oral controlled-release [10], oral transmucosal [11], sublingual [12], aerosol [13], and patient-controlled analgesia (PCA) [14]. Of these, the administration of various opioids for PCA and the administration of sublingual buprenorphine are well-recognized techniques; the others are still experimental. New regional techniques such as continuous intercostal block [15], intrapleural block [16], intraperitoneal application, infiltration of surgical area [17], and continuous brachial plexus blocks have also been reported in recent literature [18, 19]. However, these techniques provide analgesia in a restricted area, and again, many of these techniques are still experimental. Despite these interesting developments, the general consensus is that pain following surgery is inadequately treated and that better techniques are necessary [20–23]. Since epidural and intrathecal opioid administration provides analgesia without affecting sensory, sympathetic, or neuromuscular function, the technique allows patients to ambulate without the risk of orthostatic hypotension or lack of coordination usually associated with parenteral opioids or epidural local anesthetics. These advantages make the technique superior to alternative methods of pain relief, particularly in high-risk patients with compromised pulmonary or cardiovascular function [24–28], grossly obese patients [29], and elderly patients [5].

In several controlled studies, epidural and intrathecal opioids have been compared to alternative methods of postoperative pain management. The technique has been found superior to intermittent intramuscular injection of opioids [5, 24, 29, 30], patient-controlled analgesia (PCA) with IV opioids [31, 32], intercostal nerve block [24], and epidural and spinal anesthesia with local anesthetics [30, 33, 34]. Epidural and intrathecal opioids have been used for treating pain following nearly all kinds of surgery below the neck [6, 35]. However, due to the risk of late-onset respiratory depression and the consequent requirement of postoperative surveillance for 12–24 hours, the technique is generally restricted to high-risk patients undergoing major surgery. Data from the Swedish follow-up survey showed that epidural opioids were most commonly used for providing analgesia following upper abdominal, thoracic, and major orthopedic surgery, while intrathecal opioids were most commonly used to provide pain relief during the following urological and orthopedic surgery [5].

In a controlled study, the effects of intramuscular and epidural morphine analgesia on postoperative ambulation and pulmonary function were compared in grossly obese patients (range 94–184 kg) undergoing weight-reducing gastroplasty. Both techniques provided adequate analgesia, confirming the belief that the proper use of intramuscular opioids can provide effective analgesia. However, intramuscular morphine doses up to seven times greater were required to provide an equianalgesic effect to epidural morphine. Consequently, patients receiving epidural morphine were more alert and mobile (table 3–1) and benefited more from physiotherapy. This contributed to an earlier recovery of their gastrointestinal function and postoperative peak expiratory flow (PEF) (figure 3–2), and fewer pulmonary complications and a two-days-shorter-hospitalization (table 3–2) [29, 30]. Similar results have been reported in a recent controlled study of patients undergoing abdominal aortic

Table 3–1. Influence of analgesia on postgastroplasty ambulation in grossly obese patients

Grade	Mobilization	Intramuscular morphine plus epidural saline (mean ± SEM, min)*	Epidural morphine plus intramuscular saline (mean ± SEM, min)*	Probability
1	Sit up on bedside (feet hanging) with assistance	403 ± 57	312 ± 25	NS
2	Sit up on bedside (feet hanging) without assistance	438 ± 80	359 ± 35	NS
3	Stand with assistance	846 ± 115	619 ± 80	NS
4	Stand without assistance	1359 ± 218	880 ± 68	$p < 0.05$
5	Walk with assistance	1741 ± 258	1116 ± 67	$p < 0.05$
6	Walk without assistance	2049 ± 330	1153 ± 66	$p < 0.05$

* Mean time (in minutes) taken from the end of operation until the patient performed the corresponding physical exercise on encouragement.
NS: not significant.
Source: [29]. (Reproduced with permission.)

surgery. Administration of 0.5–1 mg intrathecal morphine contributed to a two-days-shorter hospitalization and a significant cost saving to the patient [36].

In a study comparing epidural morphine to intramuscular narcotic and intercostal block for pain relief following gallbladder surgery, postoperative reduction in PaO_2 and peak expiratory values were most marked in patients receiving intramuscular narcotics and least marked in patients receiving epidural morphine. This suggests that patients with compromised pulmonary function might particularly benefit if postoperative analgesia were provided by epidural morphine rather than by intercostal nerve block or intramuscular narcotics [24]. In a recent well-controlled study of patients undergoing Caesarean section and lower abdominal surgery, IM meperidine, epidural meperidine, and epidural bupivacaine were compared as regards postoperative analgesia and ambulation. Epidural meperidine and bupivacaine were superior to intramuscular meperidine (figure 3–3). However, patients receiving epidural meperidine ambulated earlier [30].

More comparative cost-benefit studies are necessary to appreciate the full potential of epidural opioids as compared to alternative techniques of pain relief.

Traumatic Pain

Few studies examine the administration of intraspinal opioids for the treatment of traumatic pain. The technique has been used to treat pain due to multiple rib fractures [37] and in ICU patients with multiple injuries [38]. The most common technique of providing analgesia in the latter group of patients who require mechanical ventilation is intermittent IV injection of opioids. In addition to their well-known disadvantages, these drugs may be inadequate even

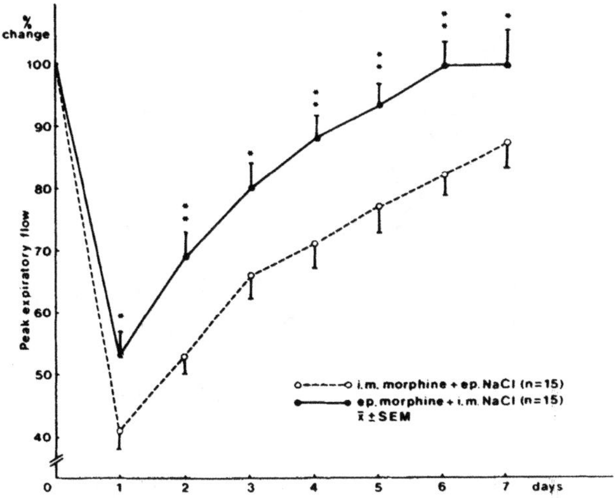

Figure 3–2. Influence of IM and epidural morphine analgesia on postoperative peak expiratory flow (PEF) changes in grossly obese patients. Recovery of PEF occurs two days earlier in patients receiving epidural morphine.
Source: Rawal N et al. 1984. Anesth Analg 63:583–592 [29]. (Reproduced with permission.)

in large doses, and muscle relaxants may be required for patient-respirator coordination [39]. Furthermore IV narcotics may lead to hypotension in these hemodynamically unstable patients. Epidural and intrathecal morphine analgesia was evaluated in an uncontrolled study of 24 ICU patients requiring ventilation due to either multiple injuries or complications after major abdominal surgery. Morphine by both routes provided potent analgesia and good patient–respirator coordination, suggesting that pain rather than in-

Table 3–2. Effect of effective analgesia on postoperative gastrointestinal motility and hospitalization time

	Intramuscular morphine and epidural saline (mean ± SEM)	Epidural morphine and intramuscular saline (mean ± SEM)	Probability
Postoperative hospitalization time (days)	9.0 ± 0.60	7.1 ± 0.30	$p < 0.05$
Flatus (hr)	75.1 ± 3.08	56.7 ± 3.06	$p < 0.05$
Feces (hr)	92.7 ± 2.92	68.4 ± 3.51	$p < 0.05$
Postoperative gastric aspirate			
Day 1 (ml/day)	211 ± 43.9	227 ± 44 ($N = 12$)	NS
Day 2 (ml/day)	192 ± 43.2	351 ± 57.9 ($N = 12$)	$p < 0.05$
Day 3 (ml/day)	243 ± 62.8	422 ± 53.8 ($N = 12$)	$p < 0.05$

Source: [29]. (Reproduced with permission.)

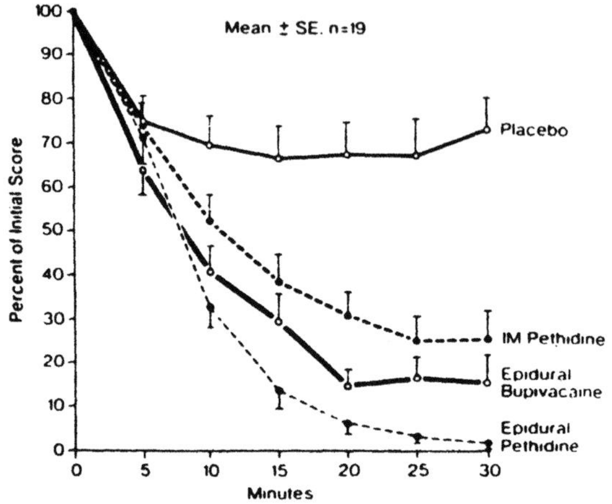

Figure 3–3. Double-blind comparison between IM meperidine (pethidine), 100 mg, epidural meperidine, 50 mg, and epidural bupivacaine, 25 mg, for pain relief following Caesarean section or lower abdominal surgery. Mean pain scores are expressed as a percentage of pretreatment scores in the first 30 minutes.
Source: Brownridge P, Frewin D. 1985. Anaesth Intensive Care 13:123–130 [30].

adequate sedation may be the main cause of restlessness, agitation, and lack of patient–respirator coordination in many ICU patients. A single injection of intrathecal morphine provided about 22 hours of effective analgesia (table 3–3). In the ICU patients, the average duration of analgesia after 4 mg epidural morphine was about five hours, considerably less than the duration following the same dose for postoperative pain; therefore, a continuous epidural morphine infusion was considered more practical. The technique was considered particularly useful for patients with head injuries, since frequent neurological assessment is possible due to the regional nature of analgesia. The individual variations in the need for pain relief in ICU patients is reflected in the daily requirement of epidural morphine doses ranging from 20–38 mg. Although these doses are large as compared to those required for postoperative pain relief, these doses are nevertheless 5–10 times less than the dose required parenterally for our ICU patients. The doses of morphine administered intrathecally are 50–100 times less than the doses required intravenously [37].

The other major indications for epidural and intrathecal opioids are the management of obstetric pain and chronic pain; these are discussed elsewhere in this book.

EPIDURAL VERSUS INTRATHECAL ROUTE OF ADMINISTRATION

The intrathecal route is a direct one since there is no dura to be penetrated and the drug is deposited close to the opioid receptors. However, the intrathecal route has not been studied as extensively as the epidural route. As in the case

Table 3–3. Intrathecal morphine in ventilated ICU patients

No.	Age/sex	Diagnosis	Duration of respirator treatment	Requirement during 24 hr before intrathecal morphine injection			Intrathecal morphine dose	Duration of analgesia after intrathecal morphine	Requirement (24 hr) of additional drugs after intrathecal morphine
				Analgesics	Sedatives				
1	20 M	Multiple trauma*	13 days	Ph 28 mg Mo 120 mg	Diaz 50 mg Dixy 35 mg	21 mg	3 mg	20 hr	Ph 2 mg Diaz 5 mg
2	24 M	Multiple trauma*	12 days	Ph 40 mg Mo 45 mg	Diaz 68 mg Dixy 30 mg	25 mg	4 mg	20 hr	Ph 3 mg Diaz 7.5 mg
3	74 M	Aortoiliac bypass	28 days	Ph 32 mg	Diaz 60 mg Chlormeth 8 g	18 mg	4 mg	23 hr	–
4	60 M	Pancreatitis	19 days	Ph 34 mg Mo 90 mg	Diaz 80 mg Dixy 60 mg Chlormeth 6 g	40 mg	4 mg	23 hr	–
5	26 M	Multiple trauma*	10 days	Ph 30 mg Mep 150 mg	Diaz 62.5 mg Chlorprom 50 mg Prometh 50 mg	30 mg	4 mg	19 hr	Ph 2 mg
6	52 M	Massive G. I. bleeding	18 days	Ph 38 mg Mo90 mg	Diaz 42.5 mg Dizy 50 mg Chlorprom 50 mg Prometh 50 mg	22 mg	3 mg	18 hr	Ph 4 mg Diaz 5 mg
7	29F	Multiple trauma*	11 days	Ph 32 mg Ket 35 mg	Diaz 55 mg Dixy 30 mg	–	4 mg	32 hr	–
8	23 M	Multiple trauma	15 days	Ph 30 mg Mo 160 mg	Diaz 67.5 mg Chlorprom 50 mg	–	4 mg	24 hr	–

* These patients also had head injuries.

Ph = phenoperidine; Mo = morphine; Mep = meperidine (pethidine); Ket = ketobemidone (an opioid equipotent with morphine); Diaz = diazepam; Dixy = dixyrazine (neuroleptic agent with antiemetic and sedative properties); Chlormeth = chlormethiozole (hypnotic, sedative); Chlorprom = chlorpromazine; Prometh = promethazine.
Source: [38]. (Reproduced with permission.)

of epidural administration, the most common opioid for intrathecal administration has been morphine [5]. There is some evidence that analgesia following intrathecal morphine is more predictable, more intense, and longer lasting than that after epidural administration. In our above-mentioned study of ICU patients with multiple trauma, intrathecal morphine provided better and more prolonged analgesia than epidural morphine [38]. Similarly, the management of labor pain is more effective with morphine injected intrathecally rather than epidurally [40]. Also, in patients undergoing open heart surgery, a single injection of morphine prior to surgery provided 17 hours of postoperative pain relief. Further, 40% of patients had even longer pain relief; no other analgesics were required during their hospital stay.

Several large studies have shown that intrathecal opioids are associated with more frequent adverse effects compared to epidural opioids [5, 6, 41]. In a recent study of post-Caesarean-section analgesia, 0.3–0.5 mg intrathecal morphine was compared to 3–5 mg epidural morphine. In 66% of patients in the epidural group, the analgesia lasted over 20 hours, while in the intrathecal group, 83% of patients had such prolonged analgesia. However, significantly more pruritus and urinary retention were noted in patients who received intrathecal morphine. Respiratory depression was not observed in either group [42]. This is also reflected in the findings of the Swedish survey. Thus, 5% of anesthesiologists considered pruritus and 13% considered urinary retention to be the major problems of epidural morphine, while three times as many anesthesiologists considered these to be major complications of intrathecal morphine analgesia [5]. The greater incidence of adverse effects with intrathecal opioids may be due to the higher CSF levels obtained. Following 0.5 mg intrathecal morphine, the CSF levels are several throusand times higher than the levels following 6 mg epidural morphine [43]. It should be noted, however, that minimal effective doses of intrathecal morphine have yet to be established. In most studies, very large doses of intrathecal morphine have been administered (0.5–15 mg).

Earlier studies used intrathecal morphine doses up to 100 times larger than those currently being used. More recent experience suggests that doses as low as 0.1–0.5 mg may provide adequate analgesia following abdominal, orthopedic, and thoracic surgery [34, 44, 45]. There is now convincing evidence that doses below 0.5 mg morphine provide excellent analgesia. Our recent controlled study showed that 0.2 mg morphine combined with intrathecal bupivacaine for Caesarean section gave good to excellent intraoperative and postoperative analgesia. The requirement of supplemental analgesics during and after surgery was significantly less in patients receiving intrathecal morphine as compared to controls. Continuous recordings of oxygen saturation by pulse oximetry showed no evidence of postoperative respiratory depression [34]. Nevertheless, even low doses of intrathecal morphine, especially in frail and high-risk patients, may be associated with delayed respiratory depression. Thus, both the 1981 and 1985 Swedish survey showed a risk of delayed respiratory depression many times higher if morphine was injected intrathecally rather than epidurally [5, 41]. In three patients in the follow-up survey, delayed respiratory depression was noted following 0.3 mg intrathecal morphine [5]. It has been speculated that hyperbaric morphine may diminish the rostral spread of morphine in CSF, and therefore may be less likely to cause less delayed respiratory depression. Indeed, despite extremely large doses (20 mg), respiratory depression was not seen by Samii et al. [46]. However, the duration of analgesia in postthoracotomy patients was significantly shorter when morphine was mixed with 5% dextrose rather than saline. The authors speculated that the addition of dextrose slows the rostral spread of morphine in CSF, thus allowing relatively more morphine molecules to bind to the lumbar opioid receptors near the site of injection and relatively few morphine molecules to reach thoracic receptors [26]. Further studies are necessary to evaluate whether this modification of the technique will lead to reduced risk of complications. In low-risk patients where surgery is planned under spinal anesthesia, the addition of a small amount of morphine (less than 0.3 mg) to provide intraoperative and prolonged postoperative pain relief appears simple and relatively safe. Clearly, more dose–response studies are necessary to identify the minimum effective analgesic doses of intrathecal opioids. Meanwhile, morphine doses above 0.5 mg appear unnecessary, since they can be expected to greatly increase the risk of complications.

WHICH DRUG?

Opioids

The choice of opioids for epidural or intrathecal administration depends on factors such as onset and duration of analgesia and the adverse effect profile. The diffusion of opioids through membranes is dictated to a large extent by their lipid solubility. Onset of analgesia correlates well with lipophilicity of the opioid. Thus, of the three most commonly used opioids, the onset of action is fastest with highly lipid-soluble fentanyl, intermediate with meperidine, and slowest with morphine, which is the least lipophilic. The duration and potency of analgesia varies for different opioids (table 3–4) and is determined by factors such as lipophilicity of the opioid, strength of its receptor binding (affinity), the intrinsic agonist activity of the opioid, the rate of dissociation of the agonist from the specific receptor sites, and the removal of opioid via blood flowing through the spinal cord.

Morphine, fentanyl, and meperidine are the opioids that have been studied most frequently for epidural and intrathecal administration, probably because most anesthesiologists are familiar with these drugs. Of these, morphine is by far the most extensively studied.

In general, these drugs have a good safety record. However, none of these drugs is completely safe (see chapter 5), and late-onset respiratory depression is a rare but dangerous risk. This has inspired may workers to try other drugs

Table 3–4. Epidural opioids: Latency and duration of analgesia

Drug	Dose (mg)	Detectable onset* (min)	Complete pain relief* (min)	Duration* (hr)
Meperidine	30–100	5–10	12–30	6 (median)
				4–20
				(6.6 ± 3.3)
Morphine	5–10		60	20
	5	23.5 ± 6	37 ± 6	18.1 ± 6.8
			60–90	12.3 ± 7.7
Methadone	5	12.5 ± 2	17 ± 3	7.2 ± 4.6
				8.7 ± 5.9
Hydromorphone	1	13 ± 4	23 ± 8	11.4 ± 5.5
Fentanyl	0.1			5.7 ± 3.7
	0.1	4–10	20	2.6–4
Diamorphine	5		9	12.4 ± 6.5
	6	5	15	2–21

* Values are in means ± SD or range.
Source: Mather LE, Raj PP. 1986. Spinal opiates in practical management of pain. (Reproduced with permission.)

in the hope of achieving the elusive goal of potent analgesia without respiratory depression. Thus, almost all opioids and many nonopioids have been administered epidurally or intrathecally. Of the opioids, buprenorphine, sufentanil, alfentanil, lofentanil, butorphanol, nalbuphine, hydromorphone, methadone, nicomorphine, phenoperidine, heroin, pentazocine, and meptazinol have been investigated [6, 47–56]. Clearly, the choice of drugs for epidural or intrathecal administration should also depend upon data excluding histological evidence of cord pathology. Preservatives, antioxidants, or other additives present in parenteral opioids are potential sources of neurotoxicity. Preservative-induced neurotoxicity has been reported in animal and clinical studies [57–61]. Focal degeneration with loss of myelin and axoplasm has been observed in spinal nerve roots of monkeys following intrathecal ketamine [62]. Histopathological changes in spinal cord have also been reported in rats receiving intrathecal ketamine [63]. In sheep, intrathecal administration of 0.075 mg/kg or 0.375 mg/kg butorphanol, as well as intrathecal injection of 7.5 μg/kg sufentanil, was associated with severe behavioral, motor, EEG, and spinal cord histopathological changes. Agitation, restlessness, vocalization, and prolonged hindlimb motor weakness were noted. Marked sedation and respiratory depression were also seen in many animals. One of nine animals in each group died due to severe respiratory depression that could not be reversed by repeated doses of naloxone. Spinal cord histological changes were dose-dependent and consisted of inflammatory cell reaction, spongiosis, and chromatolysis, Epidural administration of large doses of butorphanol was not associated with these changes, emphasizing the role of dura as an effective barrier to the deleterious effects of some opioids (Rawal et al., unpublished observations).

Therefore this author is in complete agreement with the view expressed by some workers that the administration of drugs into the spinal space is potentially very dangerous and animal toxicity studies followed by carefully controlled human studies are of vital importance prior to widespread use of newer drugs [64, 65].

Changes in the spinal cord histology have been studied with morphine [66–69], buprenorphine, clonidine, and somatostation [70, 71]. Histological examination of spinal cords in animals and man after prolonged epidural administration of morphine did not reveal any abnormalities. Similar results were reported for large doses of morphine injected intrathecally in monkeys [66]. Even inadvertent massive doses of 50–100 mg of epidural morphine [35, 72] produced no serious physiological effects other than predictable naloxone-reversible respiratory depression. Cancer patients receiving daily doses of 480 mg morphine epidurally or 60 mg intrathecally showed on evidence of any physiological or neurological changes [73]. Thus, no other opioid has been studied as extensively as morphine with regard to safety for epidural or intrathecal administration.

The choice of opioid will also depend on its adverse-effect profile. The main side effects of most spinal opioids are similar and include nausea, vomiting, sedation, pruritus, urinary retention, and delayed respiratory depression. In large studies and surveys, these are considered as relatively minor problems (see chapter 5). The exception is the occurrence of late-onset respiratory depression. This is a rare but potentially dangerous complication and has restricted widespread use of the technique. Thus, the risk of delayed respiratory depression is the main factor determining the choice of opioid.

Although the list of opioids being administered epidurally or intrathecally is long and increasing, morphine appears to be the opioid of choice for intermittent bolus injection. Morphine constitutes 80%–90% of epidural opioid analgesia [5, 6, 41]. The 1985 Swedish survey showed that of over 14,000 patients treated with epidural opioids, 96% received morphine [5]. Thus, it is not surprising that morphine has been the opioid implicated as the cause of late-onset respiratory depression. With increasing use of other opioids, reports of respiratory depression have been published [74–77]. However, because of its physiochemical properties, morphine is believed by many to be less suitable than lipid soluble opioids for epidural or intrathecal administration. The slow, passive CSF circulation carrying morphine from the injection site to the respiratory centers in the brain is believed to cause later-onset respiratory depression. Hydorphilic morphine will have very high CSF concentrations that are much higher than neuraxis concentrations. There is slow drug removal and continued rostral spread. In contrast, lipophilic opioids are believed to have higher neuraxis than CSF concentration and to have more segmentalized and less rostral spread (see chapter 1 and 2).

In general, there is a lack of studies comparing different opioids. In three recent controlled studies, epidural morphine was compared to epidural hydromorphone, epidural butorphanol, and epidural fentanyl, respectively [78–80]. In all studies, the duration of analgesia was significantly longer following morphine, while the adverse-effect profile was similar. Lipid-soluble opioids such as fentanyl and meperidine are being used increasingly out of the belief that they will not cause late-onset respiratory depression. However, this belief is not supported by clinical evidence. Several lipophilic opioids have been associated with late-onset respiratory depression (see chapter 5). Furthermore, the doses of many lipophilic opioids and the duration of analgesia they provide are similar whether these drugs are administered epidurally or parenterally. This is not the case with morphine. Thus none of the currently used opioids is completely safe.

Nonopioids

Some nonopioids are believed to produce analgesia that is mediated by opioid receptors. Recent reports have included clinical use of nonopioids such as midazolam, ketamine, somatostation, clonidine, and calcitonin [81–84]. Epidural ketamine has been proposed as an alternative to opioids because of its lack of respiratory-depressant effects. However, the anaglesia following epidural ketamine is of short duration and is associated with psychotomimetic effects in a considerable number of patients. Intrathecal administration of alpha-2-adrenergic agonists, such as clonidine, has been shown to produce analgesia in animals and man. However, adverse effects, such as bradycardia, hypotension, and disturbances of motor function, may be the limiting factors. Nevertheless, subtherapeutic doses of alpha-2-adrenergic agonists may be combined with subtherapeutic doses of epidural or intrathecal opioids to potentiate the analgeia while reducing the adverse effects of both drugs [85]. The newer peptide somatostatin is purported to have analgesic effects in animals and man. Intrathecal and interventricular administration of somatostatin was suggested to be as effective as morphine in the treatment of chronic pain. Continuous epidural administration of somatostatin has been used to provide postoperative analgesia. No serious adverse effects have been reported [86].

However, in our studies in rats we reported neuronal necrosis in the gray matter of spinal cords when doses above 20 μg somatostatin were administered intrathecally [71]. Similar results have been reported following much larger doses in rat (100 μg) [87] and cats (2 mg) [88]. That these effects may be dose-dependent is suggested by the absence of histopathological changes following intrathecal administration of 15 μg (or less) in rats (Mollenholt P. et al., unpublished observations).

Thus, although there is ample evidence that the administration of nonopioids in the epidural and intrathecal space will provide analgesia, many of these drugs are largely experimental at present. Some of these drug alone or in combination with opioids appear promising. However, neurotoxicity studies followed by controlled clinical trials are necessary before the role of epidural and intrathecal nonopioids in pain management can be established.

WHICH DOSE?

The doses of morphine for acute epidural administration have varied from 2–20 mg and for intrathecal administration from 0.1 to 20 mg [6, 75]. Dose–response studies, numerous clinical studies, and two nationwide surveys suggest that 4–5-mg doses of epidural morphine may be adequate for most types of surgery. However, patients undergoing thoracic surgery and some patients undergoing upper abdominal surgery may require larger doses. Similarly, considerably larger doses of epidural morphine may be necessary for the management of labor pain [52] (see chapter 6). The usual doses of epidural morphine (2–4 mg) that provide adequate postoperative analgesia for surgical procedures on the lower abdomen may be insufficient for good pain relief after Caesarean delivery in young, healthy patients. The usual doses for opioids other than morphine are shown in table 3–4. Except for fentanyl and meperidine, dose–response studies for epidural and intrathecal opioids are lacking.

Although intrathecal morphine in doses below 0.5 mg is effective and appears relatively safe in low-risk patients, the minimum effective analgesic dose is unclear at present. Doses around 0.2 mg appear adequate for analgesia following Caesarean section and orthopedic and urological surgery. It is doubtful that larger doses will provide better or more prolonged analgesia. They can certainly be expected to increase the risk of adverse effects, including late-onset respiratory depression.

SITE OF INJECTION AND ADDITION OF EPINEPHRINE

The site of administration or volume of injected opioids does not appear critical for the analgesic effect. The dose of morphine rather than the site of morphine injection appears important. Thus, lumbar epidural morphine appears as effective as caudal morphine for lower abdominal pain and as effective as thoracic morphine for postthoracotomy pain. There is some evidence to suggest that the risk of late-onset respiratory depression is greater if the opioid is injected at the thoracic rather than the lumbar level. The addition of epinephrine to epidural opioids does not appear to shorten the onset or prolong the duration of analgesia. It does, however, enhance the severity of adverse effects of epidural morphine [89, 90].

INTERMITTENT BOLUS INJECTION VERSUS CONTINUOUS INFUSION

Continuous epidural infusions of morphine, fentanyl, meperidine, diamorphine, sufentanil, and butorphanol have been studied recently either alone or in combination with local anesthetics [33, 91–95]. Since morphine usually provides 12–18 hours of analgesia, the infusion technique should be more suitable for the short-acting lipophilic opioids. However, continuous infusion of epidural morphine has been compared with intermittent bolus injections for postoperative pain relief in patients undergoing upper abdominal surgery. In one group, an initial bolus of 0.07 mg/kg of morphine was administered at the end of surgery and 2–5 mg of morphine was given in the epidural catheter on demand. In the other group, the initial bolus of morphine was 0.03 mg followed by infusion of 0.01% morphine at the rate of 5 ml/hr (0.5 mg/hr). Although the total dose of morphine during the 48-hour postoperative period was significantly higher in the infusion group (33 mg versus 16 mg), the average plasma levels in this group were lower than the peak plasma levels in the intermittent group. Analgesia was superior in patients receiving continuous infusion of morphine. Except for more frequent occurrence of urinary retention, the infusion technique was not associated with increased risk of respiratory depression or other adverse effects [91]. Similarly, Chrubasik and Wiemers have successfully treated postoperative pain following abdominal surgery by epidural injection of 2 mg morphine followed by continuous-plus-on-demand infusion of a 0.25% morphine solution by means of an externally worn infusion device. Their mean morphine consumption was considerably lower (7.1 ± 0.3 mg during 50 hours) than that reported by Rauck et al. [91]. No complications were noted. The authors concluded that the continuous-plus-on-demand technique provides constant analgesia in doses similar to those used for intermittent bolus injections [96].

The combination of epidural local anesthetics and opioids in the optimal doses has the potential of providing the benefits and reducing the disadvantages of both groups of drugs and appears particularly promising for the patient in labor where epidural opioids alone are generally disappointing. The addition of 50 μg fentanyl [94] or 2–3 mg butorphanol [95] to 0.25% bupivacaine has been shown to improve analgesia and favorably influence the course of labor. In patients undergoing major abdominal surgery, morphine 0.1 mg/ml, bupivacaine 0.1%, or a combination of the two drugs in the same ratios as above was administered epidurally at the rate of 3–4 ml/hr to compare postoperative pain relief. The groups that received a combination of morphine and local anesthetic and the group that received epidural morphine alone enjoyed the best analgesia. Epidural bupivacaine, epidural saline, and systemic opioids provided considerably poorer pain relief [93]. In a similar group of patients, Hjortsø et al. have demonstrated that the addition of morphine (0.5 mg/hr) to bupivacaine 0.5% (8 ml/hr) prevents regression of sensory block and provides superior analgesia compared to epidural bupivacaine alone [33].

In contrast to the practice in the United States, nurses in high-dependency units in most European countries are allowed to administer bolus injections of spinal opioids on physicians' orders. Administration of opioids by continuous epidural infusions are, therefore, considered more practical by many anesthesiologists in the United States.

Further studies are necessary to clarify the role of rapid intravascular uptake of lipid-soluble opioids, epidural fat as a drug reservior, and management and safety of top-up doses before continuous epidural opioid infusion are more widely used.

CONCLUSIONS

Administration of epidural and intrathecal opioids for the management of acute and chronic pain is well established. In spite of possible theoretical disadvantages, the predominant opioid is still morphine and the commonest route of administration is epidural rather than intrathecal. The most common indication is treatment of postoperative pain in high-risk patients undergoing major abdominal, thoracic, or orthopedic survery. Epidural and intrathecal opioids are also widely used for treating pain of malignant origin. Morphine remains the most extensively investigated opioid, but lipophilic opioids such as fentanyl and meperidine are being used increasingly. The doses of these drugs and their adverse-effect profiles are reasonably well understood. Late-onset respiratory depression continues to be a rare but significant problem. Despite their earlier promise, lipophilic opioids as a group are not yet proved to be safer than morphine, and the search for a spinal opioid that will provide analgesia without respiratory depression continues. Fortunately, recent data indicate that the risk of delayed respiratory depression following epidural morphine can be reduced considerably be avoiding well-known risk factors. However, monitoring by trained personnel and by noninvasive equipment such as pulse oximeters and apnea monitors is important. Although our knowledge about the technique has increased greatly in the last few years, many questions remain unanswered. Nevertheless, the widespread international interest in the technique promises further improvements.

REFERENCES

1. Pert CB, Synder SH. 1973. Opiate receptor: Demonstration in nervous tissue. Science 179:1947–1949.
2. Terenius L. 1973. Characteristics of the "receptor" for narcotic analgesia in synaptic plasma membrane fractions from rat brain. Acta Pharmacol Toxicol 33:337–384.
3. Yaksh TL, Rudy TA. 1976. Analgesia mediated by a direct spinal action of narcotics. Science 192:1357–1358.
4. Wang KH, Nauss LA, Thomas JE. 1979. Pain relief by intrathecally applied morphine in man. Anesthesiology 50:149–151.
5. Rawal N, Arnér S, Gustafsson LL, Alvin R. 1987. Present state of epidural and intrathecal opiate analgesia — a nationwide follow-up survey in Sweden. Br J Anaesth 59:791–799.
6. Cousins JD, Mather LE. 1984. Intrathecal and epidural administration of opioids. Anesthesiology 61:276–310.
7. Müller H, Borner U, Zierski J, Hempelmann G. 1987. Intrathecal baclofen for treatment of tetanus-induced spasticity. Anesthesiology 66:76–79.
8. Erickson DL, Blacklock JB, Michaelson M, Sperling UB, Lo JN. 1985. Control of spasticity by implantable continuous flow morphine pump. Neurosurgery 16:215–217.
9. Caplan RA, Ready LB, Olsson GL, Nessley ML. 1986. Transdermal delivery of fentanyl for postoperative pain control. Anesth Analg 65:195.
10. Slowey HF, Reynolds AD, Mapleson WW, Vickers MD. 1985. Effect of premedication with controlled-release oral morphine on postoperative pain. Anaesthesia 40:438–440.
11. Streisand JB, Hague B, Vreeswijk HV, Ho GH, Pace NL, Clissold M, Nelson P, East KA, Standley TO, Stanley TH. 1987. Oral transmucosal fentanyl premedication in children. Anesth Analg 66:S170.
12. Carl P, Crawford ME, Madsen NBB, Ravlo O, Bach V, Larsen AI. 1987. Pain relief after major abdominal surgery: A double blind controlled comparison of sublingual buprenorphine, intramuscular buprenorphine and intramuscular meperidine. Anesth Analg 66:142–146.

13. Chrubasik J, Geller E, Niv D, Zindler M. 1987. Morphine inhalation versus intravenous infusion in pain treatment after abdominal surgery. Anesth Analg 66:S29.
14. Tamsen A, Hartvig P, Fagerland C. 1982. Patient controlled analgesic therapy: Individual anlagesic demand and analgesic plasma concentrations of pethidine in postoperative pain. Clin Pharmacokinet 7:164–175.
15. Murphy DF. 1983. Continuous intercostal nerve blockade for pain relief following cholecystectomy. Br J Anaesth 55:521–524.
16. Seltzer JL, Larijain GE, Goldberg ME, Marr AT, Rocci ML. 1986. A kinetic and dynamic evaluation of intrapleural bupivacaine for subcostal incisional pain. Anesthesiology 65:A213.
17. Patel JM, Lanzaframe RJ, Williams JS, Muller BV, Hinshaw JR. 1983. The effect of incisional infiltration of bupivacaine hydrochloride upon pulmonary functions, atelectasis, and narcotic need following elective cholecystectomy. Surg Gynecol Obstet 157:338–340.
18. Raj PP, Denson DD. 1986. Prolonged analgesia techniques with local continuous brachial plexus block anesthetics. In Raj PP (ed): Practical Management of Pain. Chicago: Year Book Medical Publishers, pp. 687–700.
19. Tuominen MK, Pitkänen MT, Rosenberg PH. 1986. Continuous interscalene brachial plexus block with bupivacaine for postoperative pain relief. Anesthesiology 65:A197.
20. Scott DB. 1982. Postoperative pain relief. Reg Anaesth 7:S110–113.
21. Utting JE, Smith JM. 1979. Postoperative analgesia. Anaesthesia 34:320–322.
22. Postoperative pain. Editorial. 1978. Br Med J 2:517–518.
23. Weis O, Srivatankul K, Alloza JL, Weintraub M, Lasagna L. 1983. Attitudes of patients, house staff, and nurses toward postoperative analgesic care. Anesth Analg 62:70–74.
24. Rawal N, Sjöstrand UH, Dahlström B, Nydahl PA, Östelius J. 1982. Epidural morphine for postoperative pain relief: A comparative study with intramuscular narcotic and intercostal nerve block. Anesth Analg 61:93–98.
25. Aun C, Thomas D, St. John-Jones L, Colvin MP, Savege TM, Lewis CT. 1985. Intrathecal morphine in cardiac surgery. Eur J Anaesthesiol 2:419–426.
26. Gray JR, Fromme GA, Nauss LA, Wang JK, Duane MI. 1986. Intrathecal morphine for post-thoracotomy pain. Anesth Analg 65:873–876.
27. Hyde NH, Harrison DM. 1986. Intrathecal morphine in a parturient with cystic fibrosis. Anesth Analg 65:1357–1358.
28. Brizgys RV, Shnider SM. 1984. Hyperbaric intrathecal morphine analgesia during labor in a patient with Wolff–Parkinson–White Syndrome. Obstet Gynecol 64:445–465.
29. Rawal N, Sjöstrand U, Christoffersson E, Rydman H. Arvill A. 1984. Comparison of intramuscular and epidural morphine for postoperative analgesia in the grossly obese: Influence on postoperative ambulation and pulmonary function. Anesth Analg 63:583–592.
30. Brownridge P, Frewin D. 1985. A comparative study of techniques of postoperative analgesia following caesarean section and lower abdominal surgery. Anaesthe Intensive Care 13: 123–130.
31. Harrison DM, Sinatra RS, Morgese L, Chung JH, Mandel ALZ. 1986. Epidural and patient controlled analgesia for post-cesarean section pain relief. Anesthesiology 65:A364.
32. Purves PG, Sperring SJ, Dykes V, Stanley TD. 1987. Improved postoperative analgesia: Epidural vs patient controlled intravenous morphine. Anesth Analg 66:S143.
33. Hjortsø ND, Lund C, Mogensen T, Bigler D, Kehlet H. 1986. Epidural morphine potentiates pain relief and maintains sensory analgesia during continuous epidural bupivacaine after abdominal surgery. Anesth Analg 65:1033–1036.
34. Abouleish E, Rawal N, Fallon K, Hernandez D. 1988. Combined intrathecal morphine and bupivacaine for cesarean section. Anesth Analg 67:370–374.
35. Rawal N, Sjöstrand U, Dahlström B. 1981. Postoperative pain relief by epidural morphine. Anesth Analg 60:726–731.
36. Isacsson IJ, Weitz FI, Berry AJ, Knos GB, Venner DS. 1987. Intrathecal morphine's effect on the postoperative course of patients undergoing abdominal aortic surgery. Anesth Analg 66:S86.
37. Johnston JR, McCaughey W. 1980. Epidural morphine: A method of management of multiple fractured ribs. Anaesthesia 35:155–159.
38. Rawal N, Tandon B. 1985. Epidural and intrathecal morphine in intensive care units. Intensive Care Med 11:129–133.
39. Miller Jones CMH, Williams JH. 1980. Sedation for ventilation. Anaesthesai 35:1104–1106.

40. Abboud TK, Shnider SM, Raya JA, Grobler NM, Sadri S, Khoo SS, De Souza B, Baysinger CL, Miller F. 1984. Intrathecal administration of hyperbaric morphine for the relief of pain in labour. Br J Anaesth 56:1351–1360.
41. Gustafsson LL, Schildt B, Jacobsen KJ. 1982. Adverse effects of epidural and intrathecal opiates: Report of a nationwide study in Sweden. Br J Anaesth 54:479–486.
42. Chadwick HS, Ready LB. 1987. Comparison of intrathecal and epidural morphine sulphate for post-cesarean section analgesia. Reg Anaesth 12:40–41.
43. Nordberg G. 1984. Pharmacokinetic aspects of spinal morphine analgesia. Acta Anaesthesiol Scand Suppl 28:1.
44. Bengtsson M, Löfström JB, Merits H. 1983. Postoperative pain relief with intrathecal morphine after major hip surgery. Reg Anesth 8:139.
45. Glass PSA, Biagi B, Sischy S, Camporesi E. 1985. Analgesic action of very low dose intrathecal morphine (0.1 mg) as compared to higher doses (0.2–0.4 mg). Anesthesiology 65:A236.
46. Samii J, Chauvin M, Viars P. 1981. Postoperative spinal analgesia with morphine. Br J Anaesth 53:817–820.
47. Duckett JE, McDonnell T, Zebrowski M, Witte M. 1987. Lumbar versus thoracic continuous epidural sufentanil for postoperative analgesia after upper abdominal surgery. Anaesth Analg 66:S45.
48. Matthew EB, Henderson SK, Avram MJ, Glassenberg R, Cohen H. 1987. Epidural hydromorphine versus epidural morphine in postcesarean section analgesia. Anaesth Analg 66:S112.
49. Palacios QT, Jones MM, Tessem J, Adenwala J, Longmire S. 1987. Comparison of epidural butorphanol and morphine for analgesia after cesarean section. Anesth Analg 66:S133.
50. Chauvin M, Salbaing J, Perrin D. Leuron JC, Viars P. 1985. Clinical assessment and plasma pharmacokinetics associated with intramuscular or extradural alfentanil. Br J Anaesth 57: 886–891.
51. Bilsbach P, Rolly G. Tampubolon O. 1985. Efficacy of the extradural administration of alfentanil, buprenorphine or saline in the management of postoperative pain. Br J Anaesth 57:943–948.
52. Rao U, Campbell IT, Catley DM, Sutherst JR. 1985. Epidural meptazinol for pain relief after lower abdominal surgery. Anaesthesia 40:754–758.
53. Kalia PK, Madan R, Saksena R, Batra RK, Gode GR. 1983. Epidural pentazocine for postoperative pain relief. Anesth Analg 62:949–950.
54. Paterson GMC, McQuay HJ, Bullingham RES, Moore RA. 1984. Intradural morphine and diamorphine. Anaesthesia 39:113–117.
55. Evron S, Samueloff A, Simon A, Drenger B, Magora A. 1985. Urinary function during epidural analgesia with methadone and morphine in post-cesarean section patients. Pain 23:135–144.
56. Knape JTA. 1986. Early respiratory depression resistant to naloxone following epidural buprenorphine. Anesthesiology 64:382–384.
57. Wang BC, Hillman DE, Spielholz N, et al. 1984. Subarachnoid blockade by sodium metabisulfite. Reg Anesth 9:45.
58. Gissen AJ, Datta S, Lambert D. 1984. The chloroprocaine controversy. II. Is chloroprocaine neurotoxic? Reg Anesth 9:135.
59. Saiki JH, Thompson S, Smith F, et al. 1972. Paraplegia following intrathecal chemotherapy. Cancer 29:370
60. Craig DB, Habib GG. 1977. Flaccid paraparesis following obstetrical epidural anesthesia: Possible role of benzyl alcohol. Anesth Analg 56:219–221.
61. Feasby TE, Hahn AF, Gilbert JJ. 1983. Neurotoxicity of bacteriostatic water. N Engl J Med 308:966.
62. Brock-Utne JG, Mankowitz E, Kalhichurum S, Downing JW. 1982. Effects of intrathecal saline and ketamine with and without preservative on the spinal nerve roots of monkeys. S Afr Med J 61:360–361.
63. Ahuja BR. 1983. Analgesic effect of intrathecal ketamine in rats. Br J Anaesth 55:991–995.
64. Eisenach JC. 1988. Demonstrating safety of subarachnoid calcitonin: patients or animals. Anesth Analg 67:298.
65. Gaumann DM, Yaksh TL. 1988. Spinal administration of somatostatin in animals and

humans. Anesthesiology 69:808–810.
66. Abouleish R, Barmada MA, Nemoto EM, et al. 1981. Acute and chronic effects on intrathecal morphine in monkeys. Br J Anaesth 53:1027–1032.
67. Meier FA, Coombs DW, Saunders RL, et al. 1982. Pathologic anatomy of constant morphine infusion by intraspinal silastic catheter. Anesthesiology 57:A206.
68. Yaksh TL. 1981. Spinal opiate analgesia: Characteristics and principles of action. Pain 11: 293–346.
69. King FG, Baxter AD, Mathieson G. 1984. Tissue reaction of morphine applied to the epidural space of dogs. Can Anaesth Soc J 31:268–271.
70. Gordh T, Post C, Olsson Y. 1986. Evaluation of the toxicity of subarachnoid clonidine, guanfacine and a substance P-antagonist on rat spinal cord and nerve roots: Light and electron microscopic observations after chronic intrathecal administration. Anesth Analg 65:1303–1311.
71. Mollenholt P, Post C, Rawal N, Friedman J, Hökfelt T, Paulsson I. 1988. Antinociception and neurotoxicity of intrathecal somatostatin in the rat. Pain 32:95–105.
72. Robinson SJS, Lenis S, Elliot M. 1984. Accidental epidural narcotic overdose. Can Anaesth Soc J 31:594–596.
73. Arnér S, Rawal N, Gustafsson LL. 1988. Clinical experience of long term treatment with extradural and intrathecal opioids — a nationwide survey. Acta Anaesth Scand 32:253–259.
74. Negre I, Gueneron JP, Ecoffey C, Lerron JC, Samii K. 1985. CO_2 sensitivity after epidural fentanyl. Anesthesiology 63:A507.
75. Duckett JE, McDonnell T, Zebrowski M, Witte M. 1987. Lumbar versus thoracic continuous epidural sufentanil for postoperative analgesia after upper abdominal surgery. Anesth Analg 66:S45
76. Penon C, Negré I, Ecoffey C, Gross JB, Samii K. 1986. Influence of naloxone infusion on respiratory depression following epidural alfentanil. Anesthesiology 65:A173.
77. Rawal N. 1988. Spinal opioids — clinical aspects. In Lofstrom B, Sjostrand U (eds): Monographs in Anesthesiology. Local Anesthesia and Regional Blockade, Vol. 15. Amsterdam: Elsevier Publishing B.V.
78. Matthew EB, Henderson SK, Auram MJ, Glassenberg R, Cohen H. 1987. Epidural hydromorphone versus epidural morphine for postcesarean section analgesia. Anesth Analg 66:S112.
79. Palacios QT, Jones MM, Tessem J, Adenwale J, Longmire S, Joyce TH. 1987. Comparison of epidural butorphanol and morphine for analgesia after cesarean section. Anesth Analg 66:S133.
80. Fischer R, Lubenow T, Liceaga A, McCarthy RJ, Ivankovich AD. 1987. A comparison of continuous epidural narcotic/local anesthetic mixtures for postoperative analgesia. Anesth Analg 66:S56.
81. Bion JF. 1984. Intrathecal ketamine for way surgery. A preliminary study under field conditions. Anaesthesia 39:1023–1028.
82. Carli P, Ecoffey C, Chrubasik J, Bendabed M, Gross JB, Samii K. 1986. Spread of analgesia and ventilatory response to CO_2 following epidural somatostatin. Anesthesiology 65:A216.
83. Coombs DW, Sanders R, Lachance D. 1985. Intrathecal morphine tolerance: Use of intrathecal clonidine, DADLE, and intraventricular morphine: A representative case and review. Anesthesiology 62:216–221.
84. Mirelles FS, Lopez-Soriano F, Perez D, Lopez-Rodriguez F, Puig MM. 1986. Subarachnoid administration of calcitonin produces postoperative analgesia. Anesthesiology 65:A199.
85. Yaksh TL. 1983. The principles behind the use of spinal narcotics. In Clinics in Anesthesiology. Philadelphia: W.B. Saunders Company, pp. 219–232.
86. Chrubasik J, Meynadier J, Scherperell P, Wunch E. 1985. The effect of epidural somatostatin on postoperative pain. Anesth Analg 4:1085–1088.
87. Gaumann D, Yaksh TL. 1988. Intrathecal somatostatin in rats: antinociception only in the presence of toxic effects. Anesthesiology 68:733–742.
88. Gaumann D, Yaksh TL, Post C, Wilcox GL, Pierce M, Rodriguez M. In Press. Intrathecal somatostatin in cat and mouse. Studies on pain, motor behavior and morphology. Anesth Analg.
89. Bromage PR, Camporesi EM, Durant PA, Nielsen CH. 1983. Influence of epinephrine as an adjunct to epidural morphine. Anesthesiology 58:257–262.
90. Parker EO. Brookshire GL, Bartel SJ, Menard RG, Culverhouse ED, Ault LC. 1985. Effects

of epinephrine on epidural fentanyl, sufentanil and hydromorphone for postoperative analgesia. Anesthesiology 63:A235.
91. Rauck R, Knarr D. Denson R, Raj P. 1986. Comparison of the efficacy of epidural morphine given by intermittent injection or continuous infusions for the management of postoperative pain. Anesthesiology 65:A201.
92. Raj PP, Knarr D, Vigdorth E, Gregg R, Denson D, Hopson CN. 1985. Comparative study of continuous epidural infusions versus systemic analgesics for postoperative pain relief. Anesthesiology 63:A238.
93. Cullen ML, Staren ED, El-Ganzouri A, Logas WG, Ivankovich AD, Economou SG. 1985. Continuous epidural infusion for analgesia after major abdominal operations: A randomized prospective, double blind study. Surgery 98:718–728.
94. Cohen SE, Tan S, Albright GA, Halpern J. 1986. Epidural fentanyl/bupivacaine combinations for labor analgesics. Effect of varying doses. Anesthesiology 65:A368.
95. Naulty JS, Malinow A, Hunt CO, Hausheer J, Datta S, Lema MJ, Ostheimer GW. 1986. Epidural butorphanol–bupivacaine for analgesia during labor and delivery. Anesthesiology 65:A369.
96. Chrubasik J, Wiemers K. 1985. Contrinuous-plus-on demand epidural infusion of morphine for postoperative pain relief by means of a small externally worn device. Anesthesiology 65:263–267.

4. PERIOPERATIVE STRESS REDUCTION WITH INTRASPINAL OPIOIDS

MARK YEAGER

Progress in the care of surgical patients depends upon medical advancements that ultimately favor the development of new operative techniques. Nineteenth-century surgeons awaited the advent of modern anesthesia and antiseptic techniques, while twentieth-century surgeons had the advantages of blood typing, antibiotics, and hemodynamic monitoring techniques before devising the array of diagnostic and therapeutic procedures commonly, and safely, employed today. Throughout this evolutionary period, physicians have also recognized that postoperative care, with a less spectacular phylogeny, is nonetheless one of the most important determinants of overall operative outcome. Surgeons have always appreciated that of their patients who die from a major operation, most will die after the operation and not in the operating theater itself. It is the physiologic consequences of an operation that are frequently more dangerous than the procedure itself.

Among the known consequences of an operation is an almost stereotypic acute reaction of the neuroendocrine system commonly referred to as the *stress response*. Coincident with, and partly a consequence of, the stress response are a series of physiologic events that tend to impair postoperative organ system function. Surgical shock, described at the turn of the twentieth century, la maladie postoperatoire of Leriche, and the multisystem failure of today's intensive care unit are all different expressions for the same set of neuroendocrine and physiologic reactions that may occur subsequent to trauma or surgery.

Early in this century a prominent Cleveland surgeon developed and promulgated a new anesthetic technique designed to reduce postoperative morbidity. Dr. George Crile utilized an anesthetic technique consisting of a combination of local anesthetic infiltration of the surgical wound and light general anesthesia with nitrous oxide during the operation. Postoperatively he advocated prolonged neural blockade with neurolytic agents. The results of his clinical and laboratory investigations were published in 1910 in a monograph entitled *Anoci-Association* in which he presents evidence of the efficacy of his technique. More recent studies, many of them completed and published since 1970, have examined the physiology of various anesthetic techniques and their ability to modify some of the deleterious sequelae of surgery. Two important aspects of this research as they relate to the use of spinal narcotics will be discussed in this chapter. The first is the evaluation of neuroendocrine homeostasis in the perioperative period and how anesthetic agents and techniques modify the usual response of this system to surgery. The second is the effect of anesthetic interventions on perioperative morbidity and outcome. Prior and ongoing research has shown that the use of spinal narcotics affects both of these events.

DEFINITION OF STRESS

Clearly we will not arrive at a precise or a universal definition of perioperative stress. However, any physician who cares for surgical patients understands that the operative day and the days that follow are physiologically different from the day preceding surgery. This is at least partly because anesthesia and surgery are accompanied by perturbations in neuroendocrine and metabolic function that include a rapid and frequently sustained increase in the plasma concentrations of glucose, cortisol, catecholamines, cyclic AMP, antidiuretic hormone, and growth hormone, and a functional suppression of insulin activity [1]. During periods of maximal stress, the plasma levels of some of these hormones may reach remarkable levels [2]. Most students of this response consider that it is composed functionally of at least three components: an afferent limb consisting of neural as well as circulating signals, a central integrative component, and an efferent neuroendocrine effector limb. One or more components of the latter is usually measured to determine the magnitude of the stress response. Research that evaluates these alterations is more and more evident in the critical care and anesthesia literature as we begin to understand that the limitations to survival in the surgical intensive care unit ultimately depend on our ability to control this endocrine/metabolic wildfire [3].

The second major component of perioperative stress, already alluded to, is due to the physical and physiologic effects of a surgical procedure. Major surgery involves disruption, excision, manipulation, and suturing of tissues, frequently accompanied by fluid shifts, alterations in body temperature, compression of organs, depressed consciousness, etc. Well-described alterations in various organ functions, such as decrease in functional residual capacity of the lungs and an increase in the A-aD02 gradient with anesthesia induction, postoperative decline in forced vital capacity, increase in extracellular fluid volume, and an elevation of various protein components of the blood, are examples of this aspect of perioperative stress. All of the foregoing, and more, may be important determinants of operative outcome independent of the accompanying neuroendocrine stress response. There is obviously considerable overlap between these two components of stress, some of which have a well-defined basis in pathophysiology and some of which are still poorly understood.

Finally, it is true that no one has ever proven whether the stress response, as so far defined, represents an adaptive or pathologic process. However, the magnitude of the response and the functional consequences engendered have been almost universally considered to be detrimental to patient well-being. The goal of perioperative stress reduction is not elimination of all homeostatic reflexes but maintenance of perioperative stress within the limits of tolerance of the individual patient.

INTERPRETATION OF LITERATURE

In evaluating the literature that continues to accumulate on perioperative stress, one should be particularly cognizant of the following:

1. *Patient population.* The results of any study that examines perioperative stress reduction will be predetermined, to some extent, by the patient population under consideration. For example, if one wished to compare the effects of regional versus general anesthesia on the incidence of postoperative pneumonia in all patients undergoing elective tubal ligation, the results would likely indicate no difference. This is not a patient population at high risk for pneumonia. On the othe hand, a similar study in elderly patients undergoing thoracotomy or upper abdominal surgery would be more likely to detect a difference between the two techniques simply due to the higher incidence of postoperative pneumonia in this patient group.
2. *Type of operation.* Although clinicians have long appreciated that some operations are more stressful than others, recent investigations have provided quantitative confirmation of this assessment. The most stressful operations from many standpoints are those involving the thorax and upper abdomen. It appears that less stress is associated with lower abdominal surgery and the least stress with surgery on the extremities and body surface.
3. *Technique of administration of spinal narcotic.* Careful consideration must be given to how the spinal narcotic or other spinally active agent was administered. For example, attempts at stress reduction after the initiation of the stress response has occurred are generally not as successful as prevention of the stress response prior to onset of the stimulus [4]. Therefore, such factors

as choice of agent, dose, and most importantly, timing of administration are critical.

Early research on stress reduction

Although the technique of continuous or intermittent administration of medications through an epidural or intrathecal catheter has been available since World War II, it is only in recent years that spinal anesthesia and analesia have been evaluated as techniques for stress reduction. The earliest of these studies utilized local anesthetics to provide continuous analgesia during the intraoperative and postoperative period. Although it could be demonstrated that this technique offered exceptionally good pain relief, the side effects of sympathetic and occasionally motor blockade were considered too bothersome to allow the technique to be used widely [5].

At about the same time that continuous catheter techniques were being developed, Hans Selye in Montreal was organizing many years of his work on stress in animals into a large and comprehensive book entitled, simply, *Stress*. This book, and succeeding volumes, represented a dramatic compilation of research into the physiology of trauma. These parallel developments — the study of stress physiology and the development of continuous regional anesthetic techniques — were eventually united in the study of perioperative neuroendocrine stress. With the widespread use of radio-immunoassay (RIA) techniques it became possible not only to define perioperative stress from an endocrine/metabolic standpoint but also to evaluate anesthetic interventions designed to diminish stress levels. One of the earliest of such studies was conducted in 1971 by Bromage et al. [6], who evaluated the effect of epidural anesthesia and postoperative analgesia with local anesthetics on the hyperglycemic and cortisol response to surgery; the usual intraoperative and postoperative increase in glucose was significantly decreased compared to control patients. Cortisol secretion was not significantly depressed.

Since the Bromage study, it has become increasingly clear that several factors must be considered in evaluating the effects of different anesthetics on the surgical stress response. First, the particular stress hormone or marker under consideration is important. Some of these markers will be more easily suppressed than others, and most are affected by variables other than anesthesia. Antidiuretic hormone secretion, for example, may be suppressed by high-dose narcotic anesthesia [7] but will also be affected by blood volume and serum osmolarity, both of which may change during the operative period. These anesthesia-independent variables must be carefully controlled. Second, as already noted, the site of surgical trauma is important. Third, the timing of administration of spinal agents is important. Spinally administered drugs, whether narcotics or local anesthetic, are more effective in controlling the stress response when they are administered before the response is initiated than after. It is important to realize that the time interval between the initial surgical stimulus and the subsequent endocrine response may be extremely short [8].

Table 4–1. Effects of spinal narcotics on surgical stress: Endocrine/metabolic

Surgery	Effect	Agent	Reference
Urologic	Suppress intraop and early postop catechols, renin, aldosterone	Intrathecal meperidine	32
Upper abdomen	↓ plasma FFA and 3-hydroxybutyrate early postop	Epidural morphine intraop and postop	17
Upper abdomen	Suppress plasma cortisol and norepinephrine postop	Epidural morphine postop	13
Upper abdomen	Suppress plasma catecholamines and cortisol and urinary nitrogen excretion postop	Epidural morphine intraop and postop	14
Lower abdomen	Suppress plasma glucose and cortisol postop	Epidural morphine intraop and postop	11
Lower abdomen	Suppress plasma glucose and cortisol postop	Epidural diamorphine postop	33
Abdominal	Suppress plasma glucose and cortisol intraop and postop	Intrathecal diamorphine	10
Thoracotomy	Suppress plasma cortisol postop	Epidural morphine and diamorphine postop	34
Abdominal/ thoracic	Suppress urinary cortisol excretion postop	Epidural morphine postop	12

Finally, the level of neural blockade, at least with local anesthetic agents, is clearly related to the degree of stress response suppression [9]. Maximal suppression appears to occur when the level of analgesia encompasses the entire surgical site and when sympathetic blockade is high enough to include splanchic efferents.

With significant information available on local anesthetics and stress reduction, it has been an easy progression to consider spinal narcotics in the framework of stress reduction. We are only beginning to understand how the awareness of pain is expressed as a physiologic event. Hence the term *nociception* connotes only the perception of an unpleasant stimulus without denoting a clear definition of the neurologic activity involved. Our knowledge of some of the nonneuronal events that follow pain perception is more precise and forms the basis for what we have chosen to call *stress reduction*.

Endocrine/metabolic stress reduction by spinal narcotics

Several components of the endocrine/metabolic response to surgery may be affected by the use of spinal narcotics in the perioperative period. (table 4–1). The hypercortisolemia that usually accompanies surgical stress may be suppressed during abdominal surgery by the use of intrathecal opiates. Child and Kaufman [10] studied 16 patients undergoing surgery of the colon. All patients received general anesthesia with nitrous oxide, oxygen, curare, and halothane. Half of this group also received fentanyl 3 to 5 mcg/kg intravenously and half received the lipid soluble morphine analogue, diamorphine, 0.5 mg/10 kg in the intrathecal space. The group that received diamorphine had plasma cortisol concentrations that, though elevated above baseline, were significantly less than the plasma cortisol levels in the fentanyl group. This difference appeared late in the operative and early in the postoperative period. Other investigators have not been able to demonstrate a significant intraoperative effect of spinal narcotics in suppressing plasma cortisol levels [11]. These results are not necessarily contradictory, however, since all studies show a significant increase of plasma cortisol from baseline. Spinal narcotics are therefore only mildly suppressive, and they are definitely less effective than local anesthetics in the epidural or intrathecal space which can eliminate intraoperative increases in plasma cortisol [9, 11].

When utilized for postoperative pain control, however, spinal narcotics appear to be more effective in suppressing cortisol secretion as measured in both plasma [11] and urine [12]. This apparently increased effectiveness of spinal narcotics in the postoperative period may relate to a difference in the type of afferent nociceptive fibers that transmit postoperative as compared to intraoperative pain [13]. This is certainly consistent with clinical experience, since spinal narcotics are generally ineffective as the sole anesthetic agents during an operation (exception: meperidine) but quite effective in relieving perceived postoperative pain. It should also be noted that, as occurs with the intraoperative use of spinal narcotics, postoperative cortisol levels are usually only partially and not completely suppressed.

Catecholamine release in the perioperative period appears to be less readily suppressed by spinal narcotics than cortisol secretion. Rutberg et al. [13] utilized postoperative epidural bupivacaine or morphine and compared these two agents to conventional administration of parenteral narcotics for pain relief in patients undergoing cholecystectomy. They found that morphine significantly decreased plasma norepinephrine levels compared to controls. This effect was less marked than the suppression observed with bupivacaine. Plasma epinephrine concentrations, although reduced in the patients who received morphine, were not significantly different from control values. Similar results were reported by Tsuji et al. For patients undergoing gastrectomy [14]. Other investigators [15] have not found a significant reduction in total catecholamine excretion in the postoperative period when epidural narcotic analgesia was utilized.

The reason for the apparent greater suppression of the adrenocortical system by spinal narcotics is not clear. It is interesting to note that relief of pain does not correlate statistically with either the adrenocortical or the adrenergic response to surgical stress [16]. This suggests that perceived pain is not the only factor involved in activation of the stress response during the postoperative period. Since many other afferent signals impinge upon the central nervous system during this period (for example, volume shifts, temperature, fluid and electrolyte alterations, etc.), one should not expect complete suppression to occur. However, since the primary known effect of spinal narcotics is analgesia and since spinal narcotics do affect neuroendocrine release to a measurable degree, it seems likely that pain and relief of pain are important determinants of the magnitude of the measured neuroendocrine stress.

Interventions that act to attenuate the endocrine response to surgery may also affect metabolic processes under the control of the various hormones involved. In a recent study of perioperative spinal narcotics in patients undergoing cholecystectomy, adrenocortical and adrenergic response were partially suppressed by epidural morphine administered intraoperatively and for 24 postoperative hours [17]. This endocrine effect of the spinal narcotic was reflected in a partial suppression of the metabolic response to the surgery. Four hours after skin incision there was a detectable suppression of arterial blood levels of free fatty acids and 3-hydroxybutyrate in a group receiving epidural morphine compared to a control group receiving intravenous morphine for postoperative pain relief. In the study of Tsuji et al. [14], the patients who received epidural morphine had a significant postoperative reduction of urinary nitrogen excretion.

The use of epidural local anesthetics can also blunt the catecholamine response to surgery. This has been correlated in one study with a reduction in metabolic oxygen consumption [18]. Although spinal narcotics may partially suppress the catecholamine response to surgery, they have not yet been shown to lower the postoperative metabolic rate.

Finally, the effect of spinal narcotics on the endocrine control of perioperative renal function appears to be minimal. A group of patients undergoing hysterectomy under nitrous oxide/oxygen/halothane anesthesia were given either epidural morphine in saline or epidural saline intraoperatively and early in the postoperative period. [19] Epidural morphine failed to alter measured plasma and urine electrolytes, creatinine and free water clearance, or fluid balance excretion when compared to the control group, which received parenteral morphine for pain control. This was true despite the fact that epidural morphine gave better pain control. One problem with this study relates to the fact that the patients were required to report pain before receiving postoperative epidural morphine. Since it has been fairly well demonstrated that the stress response is easier to control prospectively than after it has been initiated, the question of prophylaxis against functional impairment versus recovery of function is again raised. However, a separate study demonstrated a significantly greater volume of urine output during the first 24 postoperative hours in patients receiving a continuous infusion of epidural fentanyl [16]. The patients in the latter study underwent upper abdominal surgery and were compared to a control group receiving systemic narcotics p.r.n.

Table 4–2. Consequences of surgical trauma on organ system function

Organ system	Effect
Pulmonary	↓ flows and volumes ↑ A-a DO^2, ↑ metabolic rate
Cardiovascular	↑ HR, ↑ TPR, ↑ C.O., ↑ coronary vascular resistance
Renal	↓ GFR, ↓ clearance of H_2O and solutes
Hepatic	↑ vascular resistance, ↑ hepatic blood flow
Immune	Depression cellular and humoral immunity
Endocrine/metabolic	Elevation of cortisol, catecholamines, renin, angiotensin, aldosterone growth hormone, metabolic rate

Physiologic stress reduction by spinal narcotics

The perioperative period is characterized by disruption of the normal function of every organ system. Table 4–2 summarizes some of the well-known consequences of major surgery. These events clearly represent major stresses on the body that are usually tolerated well if surgery is uncomplicated and the patient is free of preexisting disease. A large percentage of operative morbidity, however, will be the consequence of one or more of these functional organ-system abnormalities. They are each important, not only because of the isolated abnormality that may be observed but also because of their repercussions throughout the organism. For example, a significant fall in lung functional residual capacity (FRC) will often lead to a measurable degree of hypoxemia. Hypoxemia will require an increase in cardiac output in order to maintain oxygen transport. Thus a primary pulmonary abnormality (fall in FRC) becomes a significant stress on the cardiovascular system. This type of analysis implies that operative stress cannot be isolated to any one organ system and that any measurable stress will be amplified by the interdependence of all organ systems. Spinal narcotics may have a valuable role to play in this setting.

Central nervous system

Many studies have demonstrated the superiority of spinal narcotic administration over conventional p.r.n. techniques of parenteral narcotic administration for relieving postoperative pain [16, 19]. When compared in prospective, double-blind studies, patient-controlled analgesia (PCA) techniques appear to be equivalent to spinal narcotic techniques but not necessarily superior [20]. The advantage may still remain with spinal narcotic techniques, since equivalent analgesia is bought with a lower plasma concentration of narcotic, which implies less sedation. Another effect of postoperative spinal narcotic administration may be a reduction in the subsequent requirement for parenteral narcotics long after spinal narcotic administration is discontinued [20]. Again, this would imply less sedation.

Table 4–3. Effects of epidural narcotics on surgical stress: Pulmonary

Surgery	Effect	Agent	Reference
Thoracotomy	↑ * FEV_1, FVC, PEFR; ↓ PF	Morphine intraop and postop	21
Upper abdomen	↑ * PEFR; Fewer pulmonary complications	Intraop mepivicaine; postop morphine	20
Upper abdomen	↑ * FEV_1, FVC, PEFR	Fentanyl intraop and postop	16
Abdominal/thoracic	↑ * FEV_1	Intraop local; postop narcotic	35
Abdominal/thoracic	↑ * PEFR	Epidural morphine postop	25
Abdominal/thoracic	Fewer pulmonary complications	Epidural morphine postop	12,35,36

↑ * indicates return of values to preoperative control.

Sedation in the postoperative period is probably a far greater threat to patient well-being than we have realized. Although individuals vary greatly in susceptibility to the sedating effects of narcotics, we are all aware that a narcotized patient is much less able, or willing, to report symptoms that may augur any number of potentially morbid events. In addition, early ambulation has the known beneficial effect of diminishing thromboembolic complications. In view of these considerations, it is noteworthy that the use of spinal compared to parenteral narcotics has been shown to result in significantly less sedation and earlier ambulation in patients undergoing upper abdominal and thoracic surgery [16, 20].

Respiratory system

Postoperative pulmonary dysfunction is a major cause of morbidity and mortality in the surgical population. It is therefore noteworthy that the epidural administration of both local anesthetics and narcotics has been demonstrated to significantly improve several aspects of pulmonary function when compared to parenteral narcotic administration for postoperative pain relief (table 3).

Shulman et al. compared epidural vs. intravenous morphine for post-thoracotomy pain relief in a randomized double-blind study and found significantly less postoperative decrease in forced vital capacity (FVC), forced expiratory volume in one second (FEV_1), and peak expiratory flow rate (PEFR) as well as improved postoperative pain control in the group that received epidural morphine [21]. These results are similar to those reported by Welchew and Thornton in patients undergoing upper abdominal surgery [16], and by Rawal et al. [20] in another randomized double-blind study comparing epidural versus intramuscular morphine for postgastric-surgery pain relief.

The most important consideration in reviewing any of these results is the effect they may have on outcome. Many large retrospective [22] and smaller prospective [23] studies have failed to demonstrate any clear-cut benefit of regional anesthesia or spinal narcotics in preventing pulmonary complications. One notable exception is a study by Modig that reported fewer pulmonary embolic complications in a group of patients who received epidural anesthesia for hip surgery as compared to a control group of patients who did not receive thromboembolic prophylaxis [24]. We recently evaluated a group of high-risk surgical patients scheduled to receive postoperative care in the intensive care unit [12]. These patients were randomized to receive either general anesthesia intraoperatively with parenteral narcotic administration for postoperative pain control or epidural/light general anesthesia intraoperatively and postoperative epidural morphine for pain control. The group that received postoperative epidural morphine had significantly fewer pulmonary infections (1 of 28) compared to the control group (9 of 25).

The results of the above studies all seem to indicate a role for spinal narcotics in reducing the postoperative stress of pulmonary dysfunction. The nature and degree of the expected benefit will vary greatly depending upon the patient population under study and the nature of the surgical procedure. That is, the greater the anticipated stress and the less the reserve of the patient, the greater will be the expected benefit of spinal narcotic use.

Cardiovascular system

The functional status of the cardiovascular system in determining operative outcome is all-important. Any intervention that acts to improve cardiovascular function in the perioperative period is of particular importance.

There are basically two aspects of cardiovascular function that we focus upon in the perioperative period. The first is global cardiovascular performance (cardiac output, distribution of cardiac output, oxygen transport, perfusion pressures, etc.). The second is an evaluation of the determinants of myocardial oxygen supply and demand (due to the prevalence of coronary artery disease in the population). Spinal narcotics appear to have little direct effect on global cardiovascular function. If a role exists for spinal narcotics in preventing global cardiovascular morbidity in the surgical patient, it is mediated by suppression of the neuroendocrine system as described earlier in this chapter.

What are the effects of spinal narcotics on the determinants of myocardial oxygen utilization? Child and Kaufman [10] found that intrathecal diamorphine (50 mcg/kg) was more effective than intravenous fentanyl (3–5 mcg/kg) in attenuating the usual increase in heart rate after surgical incision. This effect was observed only during the first 15 minutes after incision. In the study by Torda and Pybus [25] mentioned earlier, patients undergoing abdominal or thoracic surgery were given either epidural bupivacaine or epidural morphine for relief of postoperative pain. Both agents significantly decreased heart rate, systolic arterial pressure, and diastolic arterial pressure during the 60-minute observation period. The mechanism of action of the morphine was presumably due to relief of pain, while the effect of bupivacaine probably involved sympathectomy as well. Although the significance of these findings is not yet known, there can be no doubt that postoperative hypertension and tachycardia are deleterious to the patient population at risk for myocardial ischemia. To the extent that these are relieved by spinal narcotic analgesia then these patients will be benefited.

Could the use of spinal narcotics prevent perioperative cardiovascular morbidity? There is experimental [26, 27] and clinical evidence [28] that the sympathectomy that accompanies spinal administration of local anesthetics is beneficial to the ischemic myocardium. Reiz et al. [29] demonstrated a significant reduction in intraoperative ischemic events in a group of surgical patients who received thoracic epidural/light general anesthesia for major abdominal procedures when compared to a control group of patients who received neuroleptanesthesia. In a study cited earlier [12], we found a marked diminution in the incidence of postoperative congestive heart failure in a group of patients who received EAA compared to a control group (1 of 28 versus 10 of 25 patients, respectively). Clearly, abnormal elevations in left ventricular preload were less likely in the group receiving epidural morphine for postoperative analgesia. It is not surprising that all three perioperative myocardial infarctions in this study were in the control group. It should be pointed out again that the patients in this study were all considered to be at high risk for perioperative morbidity. Similarly, reduction in left ventricular preload has been demonstrated in cardiac surgical patients when spinal narcotics are used for postoperative pain control [30].

Health care utilization and spinal narcotics

Given the current climate of health care cost containment, accountability for anesthetic interventions extends to the time or day of hospital discharge. Duration of hospitalization after major surgical procedures has not traditionally been correlated with anesthetic technique, but newer information suggests that this attitude may change (table 4–4).

In a group of patients undergoing upper abdominal surgery, the use of postoperative epdiural morphine analgesia significantly reduced the duration of hospitalization from 9 days in a control group (parenteral narcotics) to 7.1 days [20]. The reason for this reduction in hospitalization time is not clear, but factors such as fewer pulmonary complications, less sedation, and early return of bowel function were all probably important. When we looked at postoperative epidural morphine for analgesia in high-risk surgical patients [12], we found a reduction in duration of hospitalization from 15.8 days in the control group to 11.4 days in the spinal narcotic group ($p = 0.1$). Postoperative hospital cost was significantly reduced in the spinal narcotic group ($11,218) compared to the treatment group ($20,380) ($p < 0.5$). Similar results have been reported by Isaacson et al. for patients undergoing abdominal aortic surgery [31].

Table 4–4. Effects of spinal narcotics on surgical stress/recovery

Surgery	Effect	Agent	Reference
Vascular	↓ duration hospitalization	Intrathecal morphine	31
Abdominal	Improved pain control	Epidural morphine	23
Upper abdominal	↓ duration hospitalization, earlier ambulation	Epidural morphine	20
Upper abdominal/ thoracic	Less sedation	Epidural fentanyl	16
Abdominal/thoracic	↓ duration ICU stay, hospitalization, hospital cost	Epidural morphine	12,31

CONCLUSIONS

Our understanding of the events that lead to adverse outcomes from surgery continues to develop. As our capacity to treat more difficult and complex problems increases, so does the difficulty and complexity of scheduled operations. One of the most exciting spin-offs of this development is an appreciation of the impact that anesthetic management may have on ultimate surgical outcome. The proper conduct of an anesthetic is not bounded by the actual hours of the operation. It extends from the preoperative evaluation to the postoperative convalescence period.

Recent developments in the field of neuropharmacology have led to new techniques for management of surgical pain and surgical sequelae. Thoughtful investigators have attempted to align the use of spinal narcotics with a design for improved operative outcome. Even though we still lack a thorough understanding of many of the pathophysiologic events that accompany surgery, the success of this endeavor to date has been most encouraging. It appears that the future use of spinal narcotics and perioperative stress reduction techniques will be not only coincident but also interdependent.

REFERENCES

1. Kehlet H. 1982. The modifying effect of general and regional anesthesia on the endocrine–metabolic response to surgery. In Carron H, Covino BG (eds): Symposium: Influence of Anaesthetic Procedures on Surgical Sequelae. Reg Anaesth 7:S38–48.
2. Wortsman J, Frank S, Cryer P. 1984. Adrenomedullary response to maximal stress in humans. Am J Med 77:779–784.
3. McMenamy R, Birkhahn R, Oswald G, et al. 1981. Multiple system organ failure: I. The basal state. J Trauma 21:99–114.
4. Moller I, Rem J, Brandt R, et al. 1982. Effect of posttraumatic epidural analgesia on the cortisol and hyperglycaemic response to surgery. Acta Anaesth Scand 26:56–58.
5. Simpson B, Parkhouse J, Marshall R, et al. 1961. Extradural analgesia and the prevention of postoperative respiratory complications. Br J Anaesth 33:628–641.
6. Bromage P, Shibata H, Willoughby H. 1971. Influence of prolonged epidural blockade on blood sugar and cortisol responses to operations upon the upper part of the abdomen and the

thorax. Surg Gynecol Obstet:1051–1056.
7. Stanley T, Philbin D, Coggins C. 1979. Fentanyl–oxygen anaesthesia for coronary artery surgery: Cardiovascular and antidiuretic hormone response. Can Anaesth Soc J 26:168–172.
8. Gray W, Munson P. 1951. The rapidity of the adrenocorticotropic response of the pituitary to the intravenous administration of histamine. Endocrinology 48:471.
9. Engquist A, Brandt M, Fernandes A, et al. 1977. The blocking effect of epidural analgesia on the adrenocortical and hyperglycemic responses to surgery. Acta Anaesth Scand 21:330–335.
10. Child C, Kaufman L. 1985. Effect of intrathecal dismorphine on the adrenocortical, hyperglycaemic and cardiovascular responses to major colonic surgery. Br J Anaesth 57:389–393.
11. Christensen P, Brandt M, Rem J, et al. 1982. Influence of extradural morphine on the adrenocortical and hyperglycaemic response to surgery. Br J Anaesth 54:23.
12. Yeager M, Glass D, Neff R, et al. 1987. Epidural anesthesia and analgesia in high risk surgical patients. Anesthesiology 66:729–736.
13. Rutberg H, Håkanson E, Anderberg B, et al. 1984. Effects of the extradural administration of morphine, or bupivacaine, on the endocrine response to upper abdominal surgery. Br J Anaesth 56:233–238.
14. Tsuji H, Shirasaka C, Asoh T, Uchida I. 1987. Effects of epidural administration of local anaesthetics or morphine on postoperative nitrogen loss and catabolic hormones. Br J Surg 74:421–425.
15. Hjortsø NC, Christensen J, Andersen T, et al. 1985. Effects of the extradural administration of local anaesthetic agents and morphine on the urinary excretion of cortisol, catecholamines and nitrogen following abdominal surgery. Br J Anaesth 57:400–406.
16. Welchew E, Thornton J. 1982. Continuous thoracic epidural fentanyl. Anaesthesia 37: 309–316.
17. Håkanson E, Rutberg H, Jorfeldt L, et al. 1985. Effects of the extradural administration of morphine or bupivacaine on the metabolic response to upper abdominal surgery. Br J Anaesth 57:394–399.
18. Perkins F, Howe J, Stern P. 1986. Effect of postoperative epidural analgesia on resting metabolic rate (RMR) in man. Anesth Analg 65:S1–S170.
19. Jorgensen B, Andersen H, Engquist A. 1982. Influence of epidural morphine on postoperative pain, endocrine–metabolic, and renal responses to surgery. A controlled study. Acta Anaesth Scand 26:63–68.
20. Rawal N, Sjöstrand U, Christoffersson E, et al. 1984. Comparison of intramuscular and epidural morphine for postoperative analgesia in the grossly abese: Influence on postoperative ambulation and pulmonary function. Anesth Analg 63:583–592.
21. Shulman M, Sandler A, Bradley J, et al. 1984. Postthoracotomy pain and pulmonary function following epidural and systemic morphine. Anesthesiology 61:569–575.
22. Dripps R, Lamont A, Eckenhoff J. 1961. The role of anesthesia in surgical mortality. JAMA 178:261–266.
23. Hjortsø NC. 1985. A controlled study on the effect of epidural analgesia with local anesthetics and morphine on morbidity after abdominal surgery. Acta Anaesthesiol Scand 29:790–796.
24. Modig J, Borg T, Karlström G, Maripuu E, Sahlstedt B. 1983. Thromboembolism after total hip replacement: Role of epidural and general anesthesia. Anesth Analg 62:174–180.
25. Torda T, Pybus D. 1984. Extradural administration of morphine and bupivacaine. Br J Anaesth 56:141–146.
26. Vik-Mo H, Ottesen S, Renck H. 1978. Cardiac effects of thoracic epidural analgesia before and during acute coronary artery occlusion in open-chest dogs. Scand J Clin Lab Invest 38:737–746.
27. Klassen G, Bramwell R, Bromage P, et al. 1984. Effect of acute sympathectomy by epidural anesthesia on the canine coronary circulation. Anesthesiology 52:8–15.
28. Urmey W, Lambert D. 1986. Spinal anesthesia associated with reversal of myocardial ischemia. Anesth Analg 65:908–910.
29. Reiz S, Balfors E, Sorenson M, et al. 1982. Coronary hemodynamic effects of general anesthesia and surgery. In Carrol H, Covino BG (eds): Symposium: Influence of anaesthetic procedures on surgical sequelae. Reg Anaesth 7:S8–S18.
30. E1-Baz N, Goldin M. 1987. Continuous epidural infusion of morphine for pain relief after

cardiac operations. J Thorac Cardiovasc Surg 93:878–883.
31. Isaacson IJ, Weitz FI, Berry AJ, et al. 1987. Intrathecal morphine's effect on the postoperative course of patients undergoing abdominal aortic surgery. Anesth Analg 66:S1–S191.
32. Cozian A, Pinaud M, Lepage J, et al. 1986. Effect of meperidine on hemodynamics, plasma catecholamines, angiotensin I, aldosterone, and histamine concentrations in elderly men. Anesthesiology 64:815–819.
33. Cowen M, Bullingham R, Paterson G, et al. 1982. A controlled comparison of the effects of extradural diamorphine and bupivacaine on plasma glucose and plasma cortisol in postoperative patients. Anesth Analg 61:15–18.
34. Phillips D, Moore R, Bullingham R, et al. 1984. Plasma morphine concentrations and clinical effects after thoracic extradural morphine or diamorphine. Br J Anaesth 56:829–835.
35. Bromage P, Camporesi E, Chestnut D. 1980. Epidural narcotics for postoperative analgesia. Anesth Analg 59:473–480.
36. Cuschieri RJ, Morran CH, Howie JC, McArdle CS. 1987. Postoperative pain and pulmonary complications: Comparison of three analgesic regimens. Br J Surg 72:495–498.
37. Racle J, Benkhadra A, Poy J, et al. 1986. Comparative study of general and spinal anaesthesia in the elderly female patient undergoing hip surgery. Ann Fr Anesth Reanim 5:24–30.

5. ADVERSE EFFECTS OF SPINAL OPIOIDS IN ACUTE PAIN AND THEIR MANAGEMENT

NARINDER RAWAL

One of the most important goals in opioid research has been the separation of analgesia and adverse effects such as respiratory depression and dependence liability. A crucial milestone was the identification of multiple opioid receptors and the demonstration of high- and low-affinity binding sites in the brain and spinal cord. Each receptor subtype is believed to mediate specific pharmacological effects. Opioid analgesia is believed to be mediated at high-affinity μ_1 receptor sites and other pharmacological effects such as cardiovascular and respiratory depression at low-affinity μ_2 receptor sites [1]. It has also been postulated that μ-receptor agonists will decrease tidal volume while δ-receptor agonists will decrease respiratory frequency. Since the currently available opioids do not exhibit a high specificity, they are active on both receptors. Thus, analgesia and respiratory depression are dual complimentary effects involving μ and δ-receptors [2]. This suggests that pharmacological tailoring by molecular engineering may lead to the development of a drug with selective affinity to analgesic receptors. Several receptor-selective opioids including K-agonists have been evaluated in animal and human studies.

When the technique of injecting opioids in the epidural or intrathecal space was introduced into clinical practice, it was believed that the opioids, by binding to specific receptors in the spinal cord, would produce pure antinociception. Indeed, in contrast to opioids administered by other routes, spinal opioid analgesia is not associated with depression of respiration, circulation, or neural system. However, it is evident that in clinical practice, pain relief without adverse effects, particularly respiratory depression, cannot be expected from any of the currently available opioids because they activate more than one receptor type.

Epidural and intrathecal administration of opioids are known to modify urinary, respiratory, gastrointestinal, and sexual functions [3–6]. Several adverse effects have been reported in the literature. These include nausea, vomiting, somnolence, pruritus, urinary retention, cardiovascular depression, catatonia, respiratory depression, and sexual dysfunction [3–5]. Some of these effects, such as nausea, vomiting, somnolence, hypotension, and early respiratory depression, are indistinguishable from those seen after administration of opioids by other routes. These dose-related effects, therefore, appear to be systemic effects due to the rapid vascular uptake of the drugs. The three major nonsystemic adverse effects of epidural and intrathecal opioid analgesia are pruritus, urinary retention, and late-onset respiratory depression. This chapter will concentrate on these characteristic adverse effects and their management.

PRURITUS

Pruritus is considered a form of subthreshold pain due to repetitive stimuli transmitted along the unmyelinated C-fibers to substantia gelatinosa in the spinal cord and further to the sensory cortex. These pathways are common to those transmitting pain. Indeed, the gate-control theory of pain has been applied to explain the mechanism of pruritus. It is postulated that scratching, by stimulating A-δ fibers, closes the gate to impulses transmitted by C-fibers, thus relieving itch [7]. However, this is not borne out by the results of electrophysiological studies or clinical experience. Electrophysiological studies have shown that C-fiber nociceptive discharge is more readily blocked than A-δ input, suggesting that spinal opioids relieve dull pain better than sharp pain mediated by A-δ fibers. Due to the selective inhibition, analgesic doses of spinal opioids do not block surgical pain but provide good postoperative and chronic pain relief [8, 9].

It has also been proposed that a spinal reflex may be transmitted through a medullary itch center closely linked to the spinal nucleus of the trigeminal nerve. Local anesthetics may block the transmission of nerve impulses to this spinal reflex, and good results have been reported by adding a local anesthetic to intrathecal opioid [10]. However, other authors dispute these findings [11].

The reported incidence of itching following intraspinal opioids is quite variable. Figures ranging from 0% to 100% have been published in the literature. The probable reason is that if not asked specifically, the majority of patients do not complain about this complication due to its mild nature. In large series, the incidence of pruritus after epidural administration of up to 5 mg morphine is below 10% and the risk of severe, distressing itching is about 1% [5]. In a recent study of epidural alfentanil for labor pain, 94% of patients reported mild pruritus, but only on direct questioning [12]. Pruritus is usually localized to the face but may appear in the groin or may be generalized. The complication

Table 5–1. Adverse effects following extradural and intrathecal morphine. Data from a nationwide survey.

	Major problem		Minor problem		Does not occur	
	Extradural	Intrathecal	Extradural	Intrathecal	Extradural	Intrathecal
Urinary retention*	13%	38%	81%	50%	6%	12%
Pruritus	5%	14%	88%	53%	7%	33%

* Many patients had the bladder catherized as a result of the nature of surgery.
Source: [13]. (Reproduced with permission.)

has been associated with almost all opioids; however, there is a lack of comparative studies as regards the incidence and intensity of pruritus. Pregnant patients appear more at risk irrespective of the opioid administered. Also, the addition of epinephrine to epidural opioid appears to increase the risk of pruritus. Patients treated for malignant pain with epidural or intrathecal opioids for periods of weeks or months do not experience pruritus after the first or second day, presumably due to the rapid development of tolerance [5].

In earlier reports, preservatives in the opioids were believed to cause itching, but preservative-free opioids are also associated with this adverse effect. It has also been speculated that itching following intraspinal opioids may be a result of histamine release. However, this hypothesis appears unlikely since there is no other evidence of histamine release such as urticaria, bronchospasm, etc.

Data from a Swedish nationwide follow-up survey show that most anesthesiologists considered pruritus a relatively minor problem. However, in their opinion the risk is higher if morphine is administered intrathecally rather than by the epdiural route (table 5–1) [13]. Similar conclusions were drawn by Cousins and Mather in their review article [5].

In two recent retrospective studies from Canada, it has been speculated that pruritus following epidural morphine may reactivate herpes simplex in pregnant patients [14, 15]. Epdiural meperidine has also been reported to reactivate herpes [16]. Thus, several aspects of pruritus associated with spinal opioids are unclear and further research is necessary.

Both antihistaminic drugs and naloxone have been successfully used to manage pruritus. Prophylactic intravenous (IV) naloxone infusion at the rate of 5 μg/kg/hr can reduce the frequency of pruritus without reversing analgesia. [17].

URINARY RETENTION

The reported incidence of urinary retention following epidural or intrathecal opioids varies considerably [3, 5]. As reflected in the findings of the Swedish survey, it is difficult to establish the incidence of urinary retention since a majority of patients who received epidural or intrathecal opioids are high-risk patients undergoing major surgery who are usually catheterized [13].

Failure to micturate spontaneously following epidural or intrathecal opioid

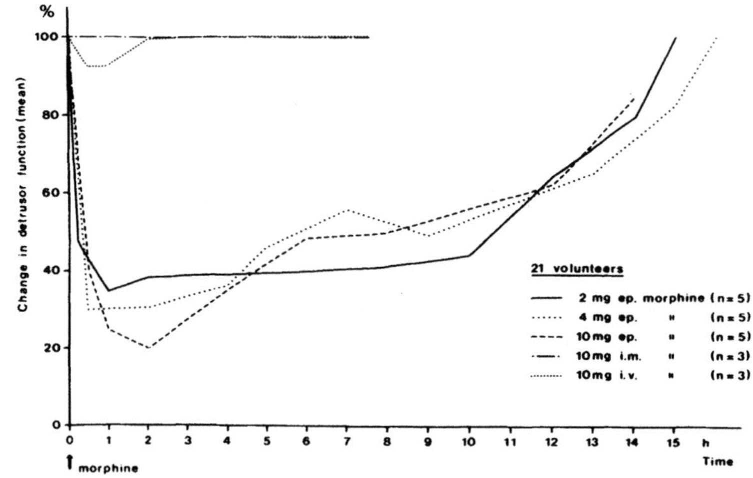

Figure 5–1. Figure showing effects of IM, IV, and different doses of epidural morphine on detrusor function: Epidural morphine decreases the strength of detrusor contraction, resulting in increased bladder capacity and urinary retention in volunteers. Detrusor function is unaffected by IM or IV morphine [3]. (Reprinted with permission.)

administration is considered to be the most distressing nonrespiratory complication of spinal opioids. This may have serious consequences if catherization leads to infection. However, in the extensive literature available there is little evidence of increased risk of urinary tract infection. Even in the infection-prone patients with terminal malignant disease, long-term treatment with epidural or intrathecal opioids has not been associated with increased risk of urinary tract infection. The Swedish follow-up survey of about 14,000 patients treated for acute pain and about 750 patients treated for cancer pain showed that only 13% of Swedish anesthesiologists consider urinary retention as a major problem associated with spinal opioid administration (table 5–1) [13, 18].

Cystometric studies in volunteers injected with epidural morphine demonstrated a reduction in the strength of the detrusor contraction, which leads to a corresponding increase in bladder capacity. These urodynamic changes are noted within 15 to 30 minutes, last an average of 15 hours after epidural injection, and are unrelated to epidural morphine dose. Intramuscular (IM) or IV morphine had no effect on the detrusor contraction, suggesting that urinary retention is not a systemic effect (figure 5–1). Since both analgesia and detrusor changes occur about 15–30 minutes after injection of epidural opioids and since the cystometric changes are naloxone-reversible, the site of action must be at opioid receptors in the spinal cord [3]. However, immunohistochemical studies have identified enkephalinlike immunoreactivity in mammalian bladder, human prostate, and seminal vesicles [19, 20]. Further, administration of

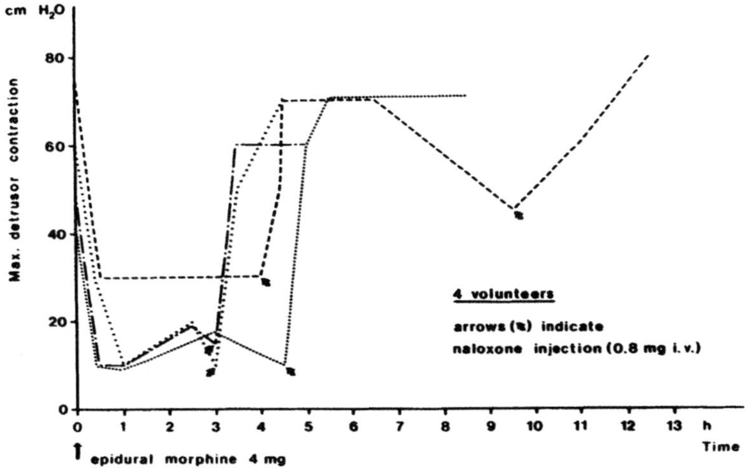

Figure 5–2. Effect of a single IV injection of naloxone on epidural morphine-induced detrusor changes. A prompt reversal of urodynamic effects is seen. Volunteers with urinary retention can now micturate [3]. (Reproduced with permission.)

IV naloxone in man yields increased detrusor pressure and a reduced bladder capacity. Since naloxone is a pure opioid antagonist with no agonist activity, endogenous opioids may play a role in the control of lower urinary tract function. Since sensory and motor activity of the lower urinary tract may be influenced by endogenous opioids, the previously accepted concept that these systems are predominantly controlled by autonomic innervation may have to be modified [21].

Some workers have speculated that urinary retention may be less likely if agonist antagonist opioids are used. In one report, epidural injection of a K-agonist opioid, pentazocine, caused no urinary retention. A similar result is reported with epidural buprenorphine. Another study comparing epidural morphine with epidural methadone for post-Caesarean section analgesia showed that urinary retention is less frequent and of shorter duration following epidural methadone [22]. In a recent study, intrathecal methadone (5 mg) was compared with intrathecal morphine (0.5 mg) for postoperative analgesia following total knee or hip replacement. Urinary retention, while less frequent following intrathecal methadone, was nevertheless noted in more than 50% of patients. The authors concluded that intrathecal morphine analgesia was superior to analgesia provided by intrathecal methadone [23]. Thus, it is clear that urodynamic studies with receptor-selective opioids are needed to identify opioids with no effect upon urinary bladder function.

Studies in both volunteers and patients found that intravenous naloxone could prevent or reverse the urodynamic changes after epidural morphine (figure 5–2). However, the usual doses of naloxone that reverse respiratory

Table 5–2. The extent of the use of extradural and intrathecal opioids for treating pain following different types of surgery. Data from a nationwide survey.

	Extradural opioids		Intrathecal opioids	
Site of surgery	Number of departments	%	Number of departments	%
Thoracic*	22	(27.7)	1	(1.1)
Upper abdominal	74	(83.1)	1	(1.1)
Lower abdominal	75	(84.3)	4	(4.5)
Hip	49	(55)	11	(12.4)
Knee	39	(43.8)	6	(6.7)
Caesarean section	12	(13.5)	–	(—)

* Thoracic surgery on a regular basis is performed in only six anaesthetic departments.
Source: [13]. (Reproduced with permission.)

depression were inadequate to reverse urinary bladder changes. Larger doses of naloxone (0.4 mg IV bolus injection followed by 10 μg/kg/hr) will usually reverse the urodynamic changes but also may partially or completely reverse analgesia [17]. It should be noted that inability to void in the postoperative period is also seen in patients not receiving spinal opioids. Voiding is also influenced by factors including increased ADH, type and anatomic site of surgery, supine position, perioperative and postoperative hypovolemia, deep sedation, etc. In some cases, the failure of naloxone to reverse urinary retention may be related to these factors. If patients are unable to void six hours after surgery and naloxone is ineffective, a single in-and-out catheterization is indicated to prevent myogenic bladder damage due to prolonged overdistention.

RESPIRATORY DEPRESSION

One of the major advantages of spinal opioid administration compared to parenteral opioids is the lack of respiratory depression. Patients with compromised respiratory and cardiac function often benefit from spinal opioid analgesia rather than intramuscular opioids [5, 24–28]. The commonest indication for using epidural opioids in Sweden was for management of postoperative pain in high-risk patients undergoing major thoracic, abdominal, or orthopedic surgery (table 5–2) [13].

Early respiratory depression and delayed respiratory depression are occasionally seen following epidural or intrathecal opioids. Early respiratory depression occurs primarily after epidural administration of opioids. The onset is within 30 to 60 minutes of injection, probably due to systemic uptake of the drug, as evidenced by plasma levels that are similar to those seen after IM or IV administration of the opioids [29, 30]. Early respiratory depression is dose-related. Due to the rapid vasculature uptake, lipid-soluble opiates can be expected to precipitate this complication more frequently than a hydrophylic agent like morphine. This risk should be increased in pregnant patients due to their highly vascular epidural space. However, in general, early-onset respiratory depression is a minor problem of epidural opioid analgesia. In contrast, late-onset respiratory depression is potentially more dangerous, since it may occur unexpectedly hours after injection of the opioid. Again, the reported incidence of this complication is variable, but about one patient per thousand can be expected to show evidence of late-onset respiratory depression [13, 30, 32]. The majority of such cases of delayed respiratory depression have occurred following morphine administered epidurally or intrathecally, perhaps because morphine is the only approved opiate. Indeed, morphine was used in over 90% of all epidural and intrathecal narcotic administrations [5, 13].

Delayed respiratory depression probably results from the rostral spread of opioids in the cerebrospinal Fluid (CSF). The plasma levels after epidural morphine are relatively low, but CSF concentrations are several hundred times higher [29]. This morphine-laden CSF reaches medullary respiratory centers by diffusion and bulk flow. On the basis of pharmacologic models proposed for epidural and intrathecal opioid transport, the risk of late-onset respiratory depression is high with morphine. In contrast, lipophilic opioids, i.e., meperidine and fentanyl, are considered safer due to segmental localization after injection such that minimal agent is available for rostral migration in the CSF [5]. Although such models contribute significantly to our understanding, they are unable to answer fundamental questions of clinical importance. If all patients are exposed to extremely high levels of morphine in the CSF, why does only one patient in about 1000–1200 experience delayed respiratory depression? Clearly factors other than high CSF opioid concentration and lipophilicity are responsible.

As a group, lipophilic opioids have several disadvantages. Their safety, both as regards respiratory depression and lack of neurotoxicity, is not fully established (see chapter 3). Results from CO_2 response studies suggest epidural administration of lipophilic drugs such as fentanyl, alfentanil, and butorphanol are just as likely to cause prolonged respiratory depression as morphine [33–35]. The quantity of epidural adipose tissue may be another factor impacting complications with lipophilic opioids. The quantity and speed of uptake of these drugs will vary with the amount of adipose tissue in the epidural space. Continued transfer of the drug from the drug depot in epidural fat may occur after use of repeated epidural doses or infusions because of the short duration of action. Also, the doses and some adverse effects of epidural and parenteral administration of some lipophilic opioids may be identical. This led Jacobson et al. to describe epidural administration of diamorphine as "an exotic method of administering a systemic opioid" [36]. Methadone and buprenorphine provide a longer duration of analgesia than many other lipophilic opioids; however, they appear to lack greater safety than morphine [37, 38]. The main

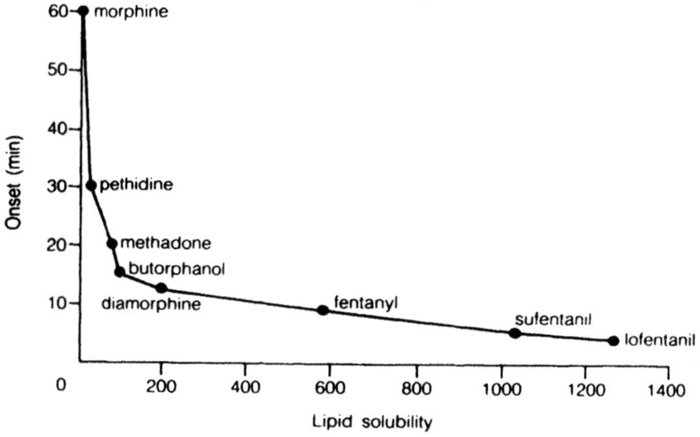

Figure 5–3. Onset times of epidural opioid analgesia against lipid solubility [42]. (Reproduced with permission.)

advantage of lipophilic opioids is the rapid onset of analgesia that they provide (figure 5–3). Drugs such as fentanyl may be used epidurally to supplement analgesia if epidural block with local anesthetics fails to provide complete surgical analgesia. Epidural infusions of lipophilic drugs either alone or in combination with dilute solutions of local anesthetic drugs appear promising but need to be studied further (see chapters 3 and 7).

Thus, it is clear that high lipid solubility of the opioid does not prevent rostral migration. Indeed, late-onset respiratory depression has been reported following epidural injection of many lipid-soluble opioids [37–39]. Our knowledge of the mechanism for late-onset respiratory depression is quite limited. The molecular size and shape of the opioid are important factors affecting diffusion across the dura and the extent of cephalad spread in the CSF. Also important are the degree of ionization, the receptor affinity and receptor dissociation of the drug, pharmacokinetics in CSF, pharmacodynamic properties of the injected opioid, and the role of sudden changes in the intrathoracic and intra-abdominal pressure due to coughing, straining, etc.

Since late-onset respiratory depression is very rare, studies involving thousands of patients are necessary for each opioid before safety can be established. At present such data are only available for morphine. Contrary to general belief, the Swedish follow-up survey revealed the epidural morphine is relatively safe. Of over 14,000 patients studied, only 13 (0.09%) showed evidence of late-onset respiratory depression (respiratory rate below 10 per minute or treatment by naloxone) [13]. A similar incidence (about 0.1%) of late-onset respiratory depression following epidural morphine has been reported in other large series [31, 32]. In Sweden, epidural morphine is used mainly to provide postoperative pain relief in high-risk patients undergoing

Table 5–3. Risk factors for late-onset respiratory depression following epidural or intrathecal morphine

- Advanced age
- High-risk patients
- Large doses of opioids
- Residual effect of general anesthesia
- Concomitant parenteral analgesics and/or sedatives
- Combination of local anesthetics and opioids epidurally

Based on data from two nationwide studies comprising 20,000 patients.

major abdominal, thoracic, or orthopedic surgery (table 5–2). It is doubtful if this safety can be matched by epidural lipophilic opioids or even by intramuscular narcotics.

The 1981 Swedish survey and a follow-up five years later identified several risk factors (table 5–3). If doses of epidural morphine are 4 mg or less (intrathecal morphine 0.2–0.8 mg), the risk of late-onset respiratory depression is greatly reduced. The equianalgesic doses of morphine for epidural and intrathecal administration have not been established. However, both surveys comprising 20,000–23,000 patients pointed out that the risk of late-onset respiratory depression is 3–4 times higher if morphine is given intrathecally rather than epidurally. None of the patients experienced respiratory depression 12 hours after epidural morphine injection. Nevertheless, *all patients receiving epidural or intrathecal opioids, irrespective of the drug, should be observed for signs of late-onset respiratory depression.* After epidural morphine use, observation for more than 12 hours after the injection appears unnecessary.

Respiratory depression following epidural or intrathecal administration of opioid agonists is easily reversed by IV naloxone. However, due to prolonged nature of respiratory depression and short half-life of IV naloxone, repeated doses or IV infusion may be necessary [17]. Respiratory depression due to epidural administration of agonist/antagonists such as buprenorphine is not antagonized effectively by naloxone; indeed no specific antagonists are available at present [40]. These patients may require ventilation until spontaneous recovery occurs.

CO_2 response studies in volunteers and clinical studies conclude that prophylaxis against respiratory depression due to epidural opioids is feasible with low-dose naloxone infusion (5 μg/kg/hr) without affecting analgesia [4, 17]. However, larger doses (10 μg/kg/hr) can be expected to partially reverse analgesia [17].

Interestingly, delayed respiratory depression occurring after a period of adequate spontaneous ventilation is not unique to epidural or intrathecal administration of opioids. Opioids administered by IV, IM, and sublingual modes have also produced this complication. Varying or decreased stimulation in the postoperative period may be responsible. Alternatively, enteral–hepatic recirculation as occurs following IV fentanyl may lead to secondary increases in plasma levels [41, 42]. Pertinent to this, a recent double-blind study comparing sublingual buprenorphine and intramuscular narcotic (ketobemidone) was abandoned due to the occurrence of late-onset respiratory depression 1.5–2.5 hours following sublingual buprenorphine in 3 out of 8 patients treated for posthysterectomy pain relief. Respiratory depression lasted several hours and could not be reversed with naloxone. Similar respiratory depression was noted following IM buprenorphine [43]. The swedish Health Board has received several similar reports. IM butorphanol has also been associated with late-onset respiratory depression.

CONCLUSIONS

Our understanding of opioid analgesia has increased greatly over the last decade; however, the goal of epidural and intrathecal opioid analgesia without adverse effects remains elusive. Late-onset respiratory depression continues to be the major problem. None of the currently available opioids are completely risk-free. However, surveys in Sweden indicate that the risks can be greatly reduced by avoiding known predisposing factors. Low-dose naloxone infusion or noninvasive monitoring (pulse oximeters, apnea monitors) show promise to improve safety of the technique, thus perhaps reducing manpower needed to adequately observe the patients.

REFERENCES

1. Ling GSF, Spiegel K, Lockhart SH, Pasternak GW. 1985. Separation of opioid analgesia from respiratory depression: Evidence for different receptor mechanisms. J Pharmacol Exp Ther 232:149–155.
2. Morin-Surun MP, Doudinot E, Gacel G, Champagnat J, Rogues BP, Denavit-Saubie M. 1984. Different effects of and opiate agonists on respiration. Eur J Pharmacol 98:235–240.
3. Rawal N, Möllefors K, Axelsson K, Lingårdh G, Widman B. 1983. An experimental study of urodynamic effects of epidural morphine and of naloxone reversal. Anesth Analg 62:641–647.
4. Rawal N, Wattwil M. 1984. Respiratory depression following epidural morphine. An experimental and clinical study. Anesth Analg 63:8–14.
5. Cousins MJ, Mather LE. 1984. Intrathecal and epidural administration of opioids. Anesthesiology 61:276–310.
6. Torda TA, Pybus DA. 1982. A comparison of four opiates for epidural analgesia. Br J Anaesth 54:291–295.
7. Cashman JN. 1984. Pruritus following spinal anaeshtesia. Anaesthesia 39:248–250.
8. Hökfelt T, Ljungdahl A, Elde R, Nilsson G, Terenius L. 1977. Immuno-histochemical analysis of peptide pathways possibly related to pain and analgesia: Enkephalin and Substance P. Proc Natl Acad Sci USA 74:3081–3085.
9. Müller H, Borner U, Stoyanov M, Hempelman G. 1982. Theoretical aspects and practical considerations concerning selective opiate analgesia. In Yaksh TL, Müller H (eds): Spinal Opiate Analgesia. Experimental and Clinical Studies. New York: Springer-Verlag, pp. 9–17.
10. Scott PV, Fishcer HBJ. 1982. Intraspinal opiates and itching: A new reflex? Br Med J 284:1015–1016.
11. Justins DM, Reynolds F. 1982. Intraspinal opiates and itching: A new reflex. Br Med J 284:104.
12. Heytens L, Cammu H, Camu F. 1987. Extradural analgesia during labour using alfentanil. Br J Anaesth 59:331–337.
13. Rawal N, Arnér S, Gustafsson LL, Allvin R. 1987. Present state of extradural and intrathecal

opioid analgesia in Sweden. A nationwide follow-up survey. Br J Anaesth 59:791–799.
14. Crone L, Clark K, Albritton W, Cronk S, Real TL. 1986. Relation between oral herpes simplex and the use of epidural morphine in obstetric patients. Proc Soc Obstet Anesth Perinat A124.
15. Douglas MJ, Thomas EE, McMorland GH, Anderson J, Cairns G. 1986. Epidemiology of HSVI infection in the puerperal population — does epidural morphine cause recrudescence? Proc Soc Obstet Anesth Perinat A125.
16. Acalovschi I, Ene V, Lörinczi E, Nicolaus F. 1986. Saddle block with pethidine for perineal operations. Br J Anaesth 58:1012–1016.
17. Rawal N, Schött U, Tandon B, Dahlström B, Inturrisi C, Sjöstrand U, Wennhager M. 1986. Influence of i.v. naloxone infusion on analgesia and untoward effects of epidural morphine. Anesthesiology 64:194–201.
18. Arnér S, Rawal N, Gustafsson LL. 1988. Clinical experience of long term treatment with extradural and intrathecal opioids — a nationwide survey. Acta Anaesthiol Scand 32: 253–259.
19. Hökfelt T, Schultzberg M, Elde R, Nilsson G, Terenius L, Said S, Goldstein M. 1978. Peptide neurons in peripheral tissues including urinary tract: Immunohistochemical studies. Acta Pharmacol Toxicol 43:79–89.
20. Vaalasti A, Linnolia I, Hernonen A. 1980. Immunohistochemical demonstration of VIP, (Met^5)-and (Len^5)-enkephalin immunoreactive nerve fibers in the human prostate and seminal vesicles. Histochemistry 66:89–98.
21. Murray KHA, Feneley RCL. 1982. Endorphins — a role in lower urinary tract function? The effect of opioid blockade on the detrusor and urethral sphincter mechanisms. Br J Urol 54:638–640.
22. Evron S, Samueloff A, Simon A, Drenger B, Magora F. 1985. Urinary function during epidural analgesia with methadone and morphine in post-cesarean section patients. Pain 23:135–144.
23. Jacobson L, Chabal C, Brody MC, Ward RJ. 1989. Intrathecal methadone 5 mg and morphine 0.5 mg for postoperative analgesia: A comparison of the efficacy, duration and side effects. Anesth Analg 68:S132.
24. Rawal N, Sjöstrand UH, Dahlström B, Nydahl PA, Östelius J. 1982. Epidural morphine for postoperative pain relief: A comparative study with intramuscular narcotic and intercostal nerve block. Anesth Analg 61:93–98.
25. Rawal N, Sjöstrand U, Christoffersson E, Rydman H, Arvill A. 1984. Comparison of intramuscular and epidural morphine for postoperative analgesia in the grossly obese: Influence on postoperative ambulation and pulmonary function. Anesth Analg 63:583–592.
26. Aun C, Thomas D, St. John-Jones L, Colvin MP, Savage TM, Lewis CT. 1985. Intrathecal morphine in cardiac surgery. Eur J Anesth 2:419–426.
27. Gray JR, Fromme GA, Nauss LA, Wang JK, Duane MI. 1986. Intrathecal morphine for post-thoracotomy pain. Anesth Analg 65:873–876.
28. Hyde NH, Harrison DM. 1986. Intrathecal morphine in a parturient with cystic fibrosis. Anesth Analg 65:1357–1358.
29. Rawal N, Sjöstrand U, Dahlström B. 1981. Postoperative pain relief by epidural morphine. Anesth Analg 60:726–731.
30. Nordberg G, Hedner T, Mellstrand T, Dahlström B. 1983. Pharmacokinetic aspects of epidural morphine analgesia. Anesthesiology 58:545–551.
31. Stenseth R, Sellevold O, Breivik H. 1985. Epidural morphine for postoperative pain: Experience with 1085 patients. Acta Anaesth Scand 29:148–156.
32. Leicht CH, Hughes SC, Dailey PA, Shnider SM, Rosen MA. 1986. Epidural morphine sulfate for analgesia after cesarean section: A prospective report of 1000 patients. Anesthesiology 65:A366.
33. Negré I, Guéneron JP, Ecoffey C, Lerron JC, Samii K. 1985. OC_2 sensitivity after epidural fentanyl. Anesthesiology 63:A507.
34. Rein P, Brothers W, Eakins K, Cooper K, Dunwiddie WC. 1985. Respiratory depressant effects of epidural butorphanol. Anesthesiology 64:A247.
35. Penon C, Negré I, Ecoffey C, Gross JB, Samii K. 1986. Influence of naloxone infusion on respiratory depression following epidural alfentanil. Anesthesiology 65:A173.
36. Jacobson L, Phillips PD, Hull CJ, Conacher ID. 1983. Extradural versus intramuscular diamorphine. A controlled study of analgesia and adverse effects in the postoperative period.

Anaesthesia 38:10–18.
37. Welch DB, Hrynaszkiewicz A. 1981. Postoperative analgesia using epidural methadone. Administration by the lumbar route for thoracic pain relief. Anaesthesia 36:1051–1054.
38. Molke Jensen F, Jensen NH, Holk IK, Ravnborg M. 1987. Prolonged and biphasic respiratory depression following epidural buprenorphine. Anaesthesia 42:470–475.
39. Rawal N. 1986. Non-nociceptive effects of intraspinal opioids and their clinical applications. In Sjöstrand UH, Rawal N: International Anesthesiology Clinics.
40. Knape JTA. 1986. Early respiratory depression resistant to naloxone following epidural buprenorphine. Anesthesiology 64:382–384.
41. Adams AP, Pybus DA. 1978. Delayed respiratory depression after use of fentanyl during anaesthesia. Br Med J 1:278–280.
42. Nilsson C, Rosberg B. 1982. Recurrence of respiratory depression following neurolept analgesia. Acta Anaesth Scand 26:240–251.
43. Thörn SE, Rawal N, Wennhager M. 1988. Prolonged respiratory depression caused by sublingual buprenorphine. Lancet i:179–180.

6. THE ROLE OF INTRASPINAL OPIOIDS IN OBSTETRICS

SAMUEL C. HUGHES

Pain relief during labor has been approached in many different ways. Current practice frequently includes some form of regional anesthesia, but obstetric anesthesia might also be achieved using systemic narcotics, sedative tranquilizers, inhalation agents, or alternative methods such as transcutaneous electrical nerve stimulation and natural childbirth according to the Lamaze method. The introduction of intraspinal narcotics to clinical practice in 1979 suggested another approach, and practitioners of obstetric anesthesia were early investigators and supporters of this new technique [1]. The initial suggestion that 2–3 mg of epidural narcotics or 1–2 mg of intrathecal narcotics could achieve solid pain relief offered obstetric anesthesiologists the exciting possibility of providing pain relief that had few maternal or neonatal side effects using these intraspinal methods [2, 3]. However, the development of this technique has not led to the "silver bullet" of pain relief in obstetric patients, because neither the effectiveness nor the complications of intraspinal narcotics are as straightforward as the early research indicated. There is, nonetheless, potential for the use of this approach in obstetric anesthesia, i.e., the modulation of the neuraxis through opiate receptors or other pain pathways that will lead to analgesia. Because this mechanism is completely different from that of local anesthetics, analgesia can be achieved without motor blockade or change in sympathetic tone. The most common side effect of regional anesthesia in obstetric patients, which is hypotension, can therefore be avoided. With no motor blockade, there also should be no negative effect upon the progress of labor. To date, the use of intraspinal narcotics has been most effective in the relief of post-Caesarean-section pain and has found its widest application in the treatment of postoperative pain. There is now extensive clinical experience in this area.

This chapter discusses the use of intraspinal narcotics to treat the pain of labor and delivery and postoperative pain. Although the application of this technique is constantly expanding, this chapter indicates the direction likely to be the future of specific modulation of the neuroaxis to achieve analgesia for the obstetric patient.

SYSTEMIC NARCOTICS IN OBSTETRICS

Before considering the use of intraspinal narcotics, a brief review of the traditional use of narcotics in obstetrics is necessary. There is no ideal narcotic for use in obstetrics. While morphine, meperidine, alphaprodine (the production of which has been discontinued by Roche Laboratories), and, more recently, fentanyl have commonly been used to achieve analgesia during the first and second stages of labor, all narcotics potentially cause maternal respiratory depression, orthostatic hypotension, nausea and vomiting, delayed gastric emptying and increased risk of aspiration, and decreased uterine activity when administered during early labor. Moreover, placental transfer of drugs occurs with all narcotics commonly used, sometimes producing newborn respiratory depression. While restricting the dosage of systemic narcotics may help to avoid many of these problems, the analgesia achieved may not be ideal. The same problems remain a concern during the postoperative application of systemic narcotics.

In general, narcotics in equianalgesic doses achieve similar pain relief, so that the choice of a narcotic in obstetrics depends upon the side effects. The most significant side effect is maternal or newborn respiratory depression. While all narcotics probably cause a comparable shift to the right of the carbon dioxide response curve, fentanyl and alphaprodine may cause a more rapid shift and a greater peak respiratory depression (figure 6–1) [4, 5]. If smaller doses of these two drugs are used, severe respiratory depression should not develop because both drugs have a short duration of action. However, maternal respiratory depression has occurred in response to very small doses of narcotics, and this must be considered when using intraspinal narcotics as well. As little as 20 mg of subcutaneous alphaprodine has caused respiratory arrest in an otherwise healthy, unmedicated patient in labor at San Francisco General Hospital [6]. To maintain alertness and adequate ventilation, the patient required the administration of very large doses of naloxone for more than seven hours. She had normal liver function and a negative toxicology screen. This patient was apparently exquisitely sensitive to narcotics. The authors emphasized "the caution one must maintain with narcotic drug usage, irrespective of the route of administration or the appropriateness of dosage." Thus, any application of narcotics, including intraspinal, is not without very real risks to any patient. In addition, the effects on the newborn cannot be disregarded and are often less

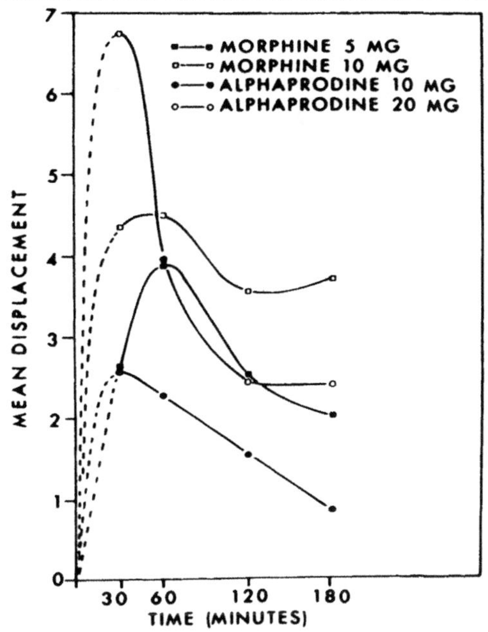

Figure 6–1. Mean displacement of respiratory response to carbon dioxide plotted at time–effect curves. Each medication was administered IM to six subjects. The initial peak effect of alphaprodine may have been missed for both doses. (Reprinted with permission from Forrest WH, Bellville JW. 1968. Respiratory effects of alphaprodine in man. Obstet Gynecol 31:61–68.)

than benign. Large doses of epidural fentanyl mixed with a local anesthetic for use in labor and both vaginal and Caesarean delivery are being advocated by some clinicians although there is minimal information on newborn outcome. This has caused appropriate concern by pediatricians and others who recognize that the care of the newborn must be considered when any narcotic is used in the mother.

The placental transfer of systemic maternal narcotics can cause significant newborn depression, as indicted by Apgar scores, acid-base status, and neurobehavioral performance. Systemic narcotics also can alter the fetal electroencephalogram, decrease respiratory movements, and decrease beat-to-beat variability in the fetal heart rate. The reader is referred to the standard texts for a review of this subject [7]. Epidural administration of narcotics to the mother achieves plasma concentrations similar to those produced by an intramuscular (IM) injection, and the placental transfer of the narcotic may lead to significant concentrations of narcotic in the newborn. Although the placental transfer of epidural morphine has been demonstrated (figure 6–2) [8], the dose of narcotic administered and epidural injection-to-delivery time are obviously of great significance. This concept is particularly important when considering

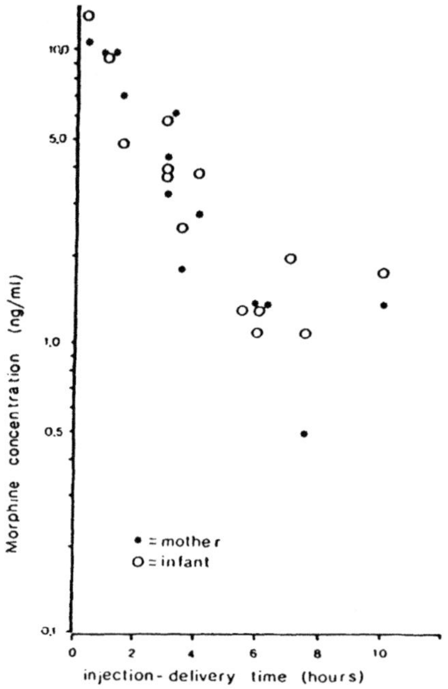

Figure 6–2. Epidural narcotics and newborn drug levels. (Reprinted with permission from Nybell-Lindahl G, Carlsson C, Ingemarsson I, Westgren M, Paalzow L. 1981. Maternal and fetal concentrations of morphine after epidural administration during labor. Am J Obstet Gynecol 139: 20–21.)

the use of epidural narcotics for the patient in labor or if epidural narcotics are to be added to the local anesthetic prior to Caesarean delivery. However, the plasma morphine levels achieved in these patients were relatively low, since 20 ng/ml is said to be the analgesic level.

Relatively few studies have explored the effects of intraspinal narcotics, other than morphine, on fetal outcome or fetal plasma narcotic concentrations. The rapid placental transfer of the synthetic narcotics alfentanil, sufentanil, and fentanyl has been demonstrated in sheep (figure 6–3), although the doses of narcotic administered in this study were much higher than those suggested for clinical practice [9]. When the awake, full-term ewe was given an intravenous (IV) bolus dose of alfentanil, 250 μg/kg, sufentanil, 5 μg/kg, or fentanyl, 24 μg/kg, plasma concentrations of narcotic in mother and fetus were similar with all three narcotics, despite the differences among these three agents in lipid solubility, degree of ionization, and protein binding.

An additional risk associated with this group of drugs is the potential of higher (possibly dangerous) narcotic concentrations in the brain compared with the plasma levels. In dogs, the high lipid content of the brain and the significant lipid solubility of fentanyl result in higher narcotic concentrations in brain (ng/g of brain tissue) than in plasma (ng/ml serum) [10]. In addition,

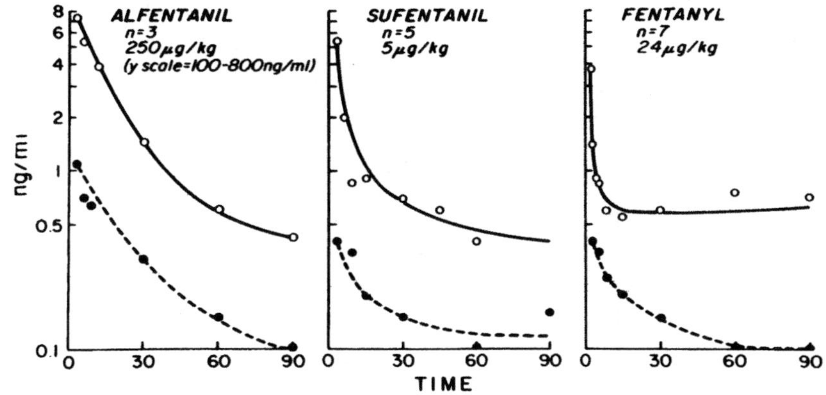

Figure 6–3.. Washout curves for maternal (solid line) and fetal (dashed line) serum narcotic concentrations following an IV bolus of alfentanil, 250 μg/kg (left panel), sufentanil, 5 μg/kg (center panel), and fentanyl, 24 μg/kg (right panel). Study was done on awake term-pregnant sheep. (Reprinted with permission from Eisele JH. 1984. The use of short acting narcotics in obstetric anesthesia and the effects on the newborn. In Estafanous FG (ed(: Opioids in Anesthesia, Chapter 18.

cerebral concentrations increase with hypocarbia in dogs (figure 6–4), suggesting the possibility of increased cerebral narcotic concentrations in humans when a parturient is hyperventilating, although this theory is highly speculative and under investigation; the possible development of decreased uterine blood flow when the parturient hyperventilates and of fetal acidosis made analysis complicated. However, narcotic concentrations in umbilical cord plasma may not reflect cerebral tissue concentrations in the newborn. Thus careful consideration of the newborn's outcome is required when lipid-soluble agents such as fentanyl or its derivatives are to be combined with local anesthetics for epidural analgesia during labor and vaginal delivery, or to be administered either intravenously or epidurally before Caesarean delivery.

Although narcotics can be administered safely to a patient during labor and delivery, either systemically or intraspinally, the potential maternal and neonatal side effects much be carefully evaluated, especially when higher epidural doses or more frequent administration schedules for narcotics are suggested. There is always a price to be paid to achieve analgesia.

LABOR AND DELIVERY

Intrathecal opiates

Having considered the general concerns and prohibitions regarding the use of narcotics in obstetrics, it is easy to understand the eagerness with which intraspinal narcotics were greated in the obstetric anesthesia community. Long-lasting pain relief with very small doses of narcotics (1–2 mg) would seem

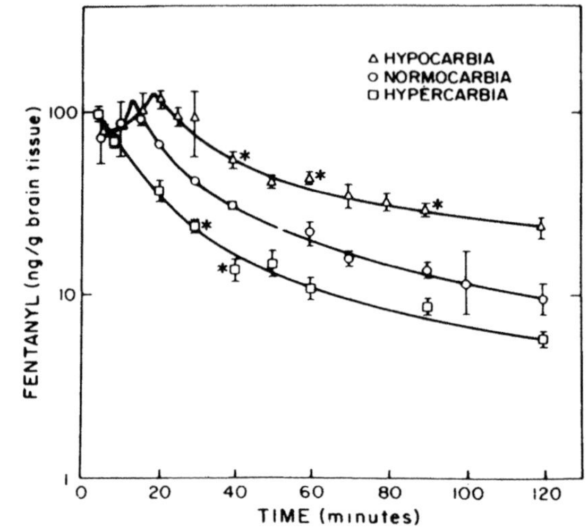

Figure 6–4. Fentanyl levels in brain measured over two hours in three groups of dogs during normocarbia, hypocarbia, and hypercarbia. * indicate significant differences ($p < 0.05$) when compared with normocarbia by the Student T-test. (Reprinted with permission From Ainslie FG, Eisele JH, Corkhill G. 1979. Fentanyl concentrations in brain and the serum during respiratory acid base changes in the dog. Anesthesiology 295–297.)

ideal for the parturient. By applying small doses of intraspinal narcotics (epidural or spinal) in proximity to the substantia gelatinosa of the dorsal horn, analgesia would be possible with fewer systemic effects and no likely effects on the fetus or newborn because the dose of narcotics suggested was small. While this has not proven completely true, to a large extent, it is possible. The intrathecal application of narcotics for labor and delivery has proven most successful thus far. Wang and coworkers demonstrated the effective and safe use of 0.5–1 mg of intrathecal morphine to treat chronic pain and suggested in this seminal work the obvious potential for the obstetric patient [2].

The first use of intrathecal morphine in obstetric patients suggested that this technique could provide good pain relief in labor [11]. Although a relatively small study, this early work made several important observations, the first being that the pain relief achieved with intraspinal narcotics was unlike that obtained with a local anesthetic. Patients "felt contractions" but were not in pain. This author's experience with epidural morphine (7.5 mg) has been similar: patients are aware of contractions, but most do not request further analgesia [12]. This effect may eventually benefit those interested in a nearly natural childbirth experience. Pain relief in the second stage of labor is variable, and if surgical manipulation is required after intrathecal or epidural narcotics, further anesthetic intervention is necessary in the form of epidural anesthesia with a local anesthetic, infiltration with a local anesthetic, or other

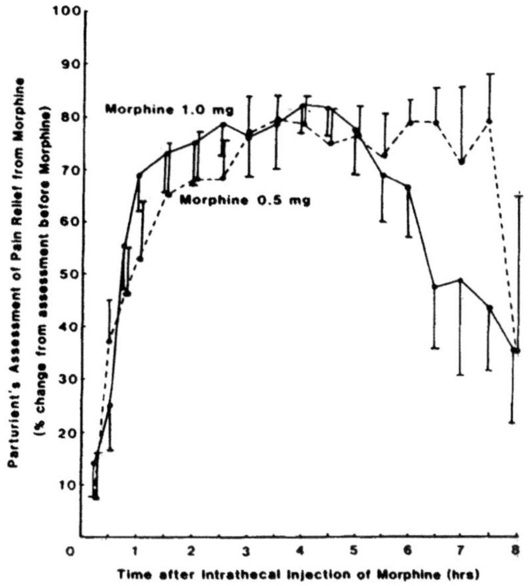

Figure 6–5. The parturient's assessment of pain relief from morphine during labor. Pain relief was achieved with 0.5 mg (N = 12) and 1.0 mg (N = 18) of intrathecal morphine in 7.5% dextrose administered when the cervix was 4–8 cm dilated. Both doses provided excellent pain relief during the first stage of labor. There were few patients remaining in the study at 6 hours. (Reprinted with permission from Abboud TK, Shnider SM, Dailey PA, Raya JA, Sarkis F, Grobler NM, Sadri S, Khoo SS, DeSousa B, Baysinger CL, Miller F. 1984. Intrathecal administration of hyperbaric morphine for the relief of pain in labour. Anaesth 56:1351–1360.)

techniques. Intraspinal narcotics cannot provide *surgical* anesthesia. For this reason, the intrathecal route of spinal administration is not as flexible as epidural administration with a catheter in place. One investigator combined the advantages of both routes by administering morphine intrathecally, then placing an epidural catheter to provide flexibility during the second stage of labor [13]. How practical this strategy might be is left to the reader.

Determining the dose

As little as 0.5 mg of intrathecal morphine has proven effective for labor analgesia when compared with 1 mg (figure 6–5) [14]. The ideal intrathecal dose is yet to be determined, but the lower doses might well be effective. In one study, as little as 0.25 mg produced significant concentrations of morphine in the cerebrospinal fluid, indicating that the opiate receptors in the dorsal horn were probably maximally saturated with morphine [15]. In patients presenting for major lower limb surgery, 0.1 mg of intrathecal morphine has been proven effective for postoperative pain [16]. Many early investigators may have been "overdosing" patients with intrathecal morphine.

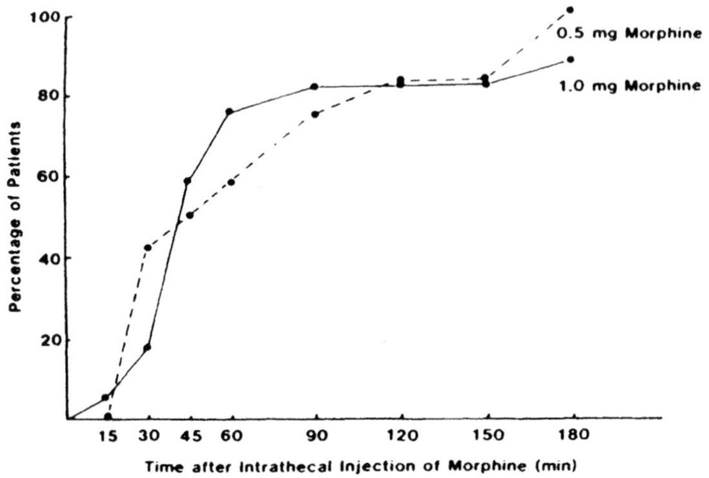

Figure 6–6. Onset of pain relief with intrathecal morphine. (The onset of epidural morphine is similar to intrathecal morphine.) (Reprinted with permission from Abboud TK, Shnider SM, Dailey PA, Raja JA, Sarkis F, Grobler NM, Sadri S, Khoo SS, DeSousa B, Baysinger CL, Miller F. 1984. Intrathecal administration of hyperbaric morphine for the relief of pain in labour. Br J Anaesth 56:1351–1360.)

Onset and duration of analgesia

One limitation to the use of intraspinal narcotics in labor is the slow onset of analgesia. Both epidural and intrathecal morphine have an onset time of approximately 30–60 minutes. The lag time appears to be due to slow neural penetration, at least with morphine. As demonstrated in figure 6–6, both 0.5 mg and 1.0 mg of intrathecal morphine have a similar slow onset, and this is not acceptable when a patient is in acute pain. Perhaps the use of more lipid-soluble agents would solve this problem. Fentanyl has been used intraspinally, but its duration of action is too brief to provide adequate relief during labor and would probably be less than ideal for postoperative pain relief. Current research suggests that intrathecal fentanyl can provide no more than four hours of postoperative pain relief. Thus, the use of the lipid-soluble agents requires further investigation.

A second approach to the problems of onset and duration would be to combine a small dose of morphine with a local anesthetic, a technique used in patients undergoing transurethral resection of the prostate. Tetracaine, 12–14 mg, was administered with 1 mg of morphine for successful relief of post-operative pain [17]. A similar technique might be successful in the obstetric patient, that is, combining a small dose of a local anesthetic for fast onset of pain relief and a small amount of morphine for long-lasting relief. Intrathecal morphine alone is not necessarily a practical strategy for routine use because of the slow onset, lack of flexibility, and expected incidence of postdural puncture headache, but it might be helpful in specific cases.

The successful management of a parturient having Wolff–Parkinson–White syndrome is a case in point. These patients are prone to arrhythmias that can be accompanied by significant hypotension, a major risk factor since both maternal and fetal well-being are dependent on a stable heart rhythm and blood pressure. The administration of 1 mg of intrathecal morphine during labor provided analgesia with minimal cardiac or hemodynamic changes (there is no sympathetic blockade with intraspinal narcotics) [18]. A vigorous 3950-g infant was delivered, and the only maternal side effect was mild pruritus that was easily treated with 0.05 mg of naloxone. The patient also required a single bladder catherization 5.5 hours after delivery, a procedure that is not uncommon for any parturient. A similarly successful application of intrathecal morphine has been reported in a parturient having cystic fibrosis and significant pulmonary disease [19].

A third approach to the problems associated with onset and duration would be to administer intrathecal morphine early in the course of labor, instead of waiting until active labor (4–5 cm cervical dilation). If the pain is blocked before it is begun, it might be more effectively controlled. This strategy might be attempted in a selected group of high-risk cardiac patients in whom it would be important to avoid the tachycardia associated with pain as well as the cardiovascular changes associated with a more routine regional anesthetic.

Future intrathecal choices

The function of the neuroaxis is complex, involving several different mechanisms in pain modulation. The clinical work to date has focused on the role of opiate receptors; however, the future is wide open. In animals, intrathecal clonidine, an alpha-2 adrenergic agonist, produces analgesia in a dose-dependent manner (figure 6–7) [20] by an opiate-independent mechanism [21]. In humans, the experimental application of 0.3 mg of intrathecal clonidine has produced significant relief from chronic pain, but has result in hypotension and sedation, effects which are undesirable in the obstetric patient. In a recent sheep protocol, epidural clonidine was effective without producing hypotension, respiratory depression, or neurotoxicity [22]. This demonstrates that the adrenergic receptors are involved in the production of analgesia. Epinephrine alone, for example, will suppress noxious stimuli and, when administered intraspinally with a local anesthetic, will improve analgesia [23].

Other intrathecal agents activating nonopiate pathways have been used to decrease pain with some success. Intrathecal ketamine, 50 mg, with 5% dextrose and 0.1 mg of epinephrine can produce surgical anesthesia lasting one hour [24]. However, in a study of rats given 200 to 1600 μg/kg of intrathecal ketamine or 1 μg/kg of morphine, better analgesia was achieved with morphine [25]. Moreover, three of the rats given ketamine died shortly after injection of this agent. Histopathological examination of the spinal cords and

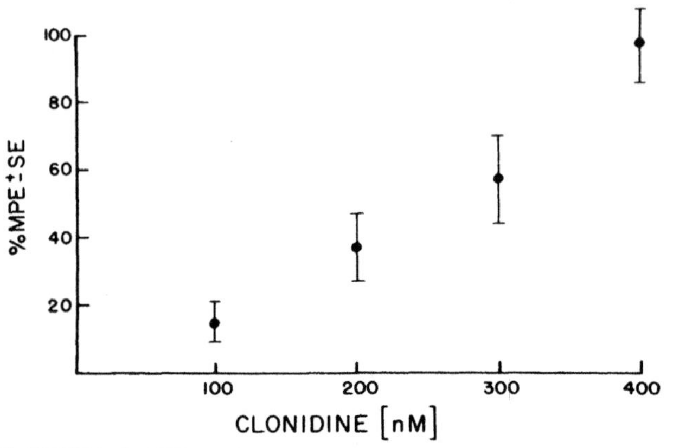

Figure 6–7. Effect of intrathecal clonidine on tail-flick analgesia:

$$\% \text{ MPE} = \frac{\text{Postdrug latency} - \text{baseline(s)}}{\text{Cut-off time} - \text{baseline(s)}} \times 100$$

Rats achieved increasing analgesia from intrathecal clonidine (an α–2 adrenergic agonist) administraion. Similar effects have been demonstrated with epinephrine administration. (Reprinted with permission from Milne B, Cervenko FW, Jhamandas K, Sutak M. 1985. Intrathecal clonidine: Analgesia and effect on opiate withdrawal in the rat. Anesthesiology 62:34–38.)

nerve roots in these three rats revealed vacuoles in the cells of the posterior root ganglion. The issue of neurotoxicity was investigated in monkeys, and focal degeneration with loss of myelin and axoplasm was observed in two monkeys who had received ketamine [26]. Consequently, reports of the successful use of ketamine as an intraspinal agent should be reviewed with care until the question of this drug's neurotoxicity is resolved.

One recent study also demonstrated profound postoperative analgesia using intrathecal salmon calcitonin (100 I.U.) [27]. Calcitonin is a polypeptide found in the thyroid, brain, pituitary, and cerebrospinal fluid, but its physiologic function is not fully defined. Although its effects on calcium and phosphate metabolism are well known, it produces prolonged analgesia in humans and animals by an unknown mechanism. The clinical relevance of these studies to general pain relief, such as severe chronic pain, let alone elective obstetric analgesia, remains unclear.

The possibility of useful modulation of the neuroaxis with drugs other than opiates seems likely, but is unproven at present. Caution is necessary before using any new drugs as intrathecal agents. There may be clinical side effects of any new approach that are not immediately obvious. For example, the risk of direct neurologic toxicity must be carefully examined. In one laboratory report, the narcotic piritramide (pH 3.38–3.96) was thought to cause deproteinization in the CSF and therefore to be inappropriate for intraspinal use. Surprisingly, opium also may be contraindicated for intrathecal use [28].

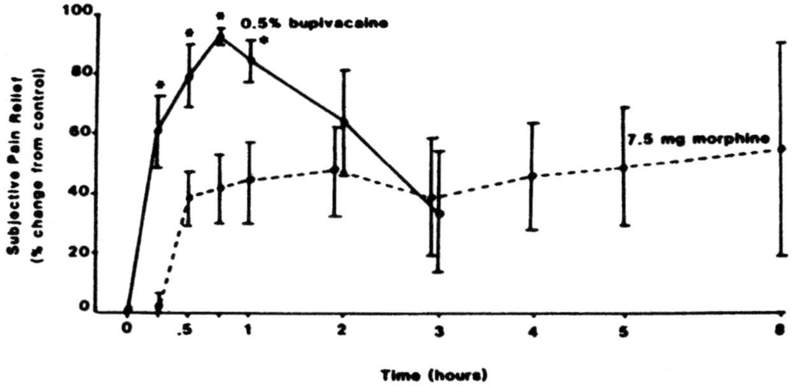

Figure 6–8. Subjective pain relief calculated from the visual linear analogue scale (mean ± SEM) contrasting 0.5% epidural bupivacaine with 7.5 mg epidural morphine over time. * indicates a significant difference ($p < 0.01$). The 2 mg and 5 mg doses of epidural morphine were ineffective. (Reprinted by permission from the International Anesthesia Research Society from Hughes SC, Rosen MA, Shnider SM, Abboud TK, Stefani SJ, Norton M. 1984. Maternal and neonatal effects of epidural morphine for labor and delivery. Anesth Analg 63:319–324.)

While the use of new approaches to pain relief are fascinating, a thoughtful, logical approach is necessary. However, intrathecal morphine remains a viable alternative for analgesia during labor and delivery in selected obstetric patients. While the side effects of this method (chapter 5) demand increased attention, the pain relief provided is excellent and the benefits make it a worthwhile approach in some patients.

Epidural opioids

The use of epidural analgesia and anesthesia in the obstetric suite is well established. When Behar et al. published a report of the successful use of 2 mg of epidural morphine for patients in chronic pain, the application of obstetric anesthesia seemed an obvious alternative and many scientists began to investigate this new approach. Husemeyer et al. tried 2 mg of preservative-free epidural morphine for labor and found that the pain relief was inadequate [29]. Their results were confirmed by this author and his coworkers, who applied slightly higher doses of morphine (2.5–7.5 mg) and compared epidural morphine to 0.5% bupivacaine. Other investigators using 2–5 mg of epidural morphine also found these doses inadequate [30–32]. The question at that point was why as little as 0.5 mg of intrathecal morphine could achieve pain relief and yet epidural morphine in much higher doses could not. Moreover, why was the treatment of chronic pain and postoperative pain using small doses of epidural morphine so successful and analgesia for labor so inadequate? What is the nature of labor pain? The answer to this last question is still unclear, but our work suggested a dose response with epidural morphine to

Table 6–1. Intraspinal morphine and CSF concentration*

Site of administration and dose	Concentration (time after administration)	
	1hr	18hr
Epidural, 2–6 mg	200–1,000 ng/ml	25–40 ng/ml
Spinal, 0.25–0.50 mg	4,000–10,000 ng/ml	180–200 ng/ml

* Adapted from Nordberg G, Hedner T, Mellstrand T, Dahlström B. 1984. Pharmacokinetic aspects of intrathecal morphine analgesia. Anesthesiology 60:448–454. (Reprinted with permission from Hughes SC. 1987. Intraspinal opiates in obstetrics. In Shnider SM, Levinson G (eds): Anesthesia for Obstetrics. Philadelphia: Williams and Wilkins, Chapter 10.)

treat the pain of labor and delivery [12]. That is, we demonstrated that 2.5 mg and 5 mg of epidural morphine were ineffective, but that 7.5 mg provided adequate pain relief for some patients (figure 6–8). Although the analgesia produced was not as solid as that achieved in a control group given bupivacaine, 0.5% (a surgical anesthetic that is rarely, if ever, used in this author's practice today for labor analgesia), it was similar to that obtained in the patients mentioned earlier who had received a low dose of intrathecal morphine, and "felt contractions," but required no further medication. Research on the pharmacokinetic aspects of intraspinal narcotics has demonstrated that very small doses of intrathecal narcotics will achieve very high concentrations of the drug in the CSF, while epidural doses must be 10–20 times higher than an intrathecal dose to achieve a similar CSF concentration (table 6–1). Doses of 7.5 mg of epidural morphine *or more* seem to be needed for labor analgesia. Epidural morphine, 10 mg, has been used in labor with mixed results and significant side effects of nausea, vomiting, and drowsiness [33, 34]. As previously discussed, concern for the newborn rises as well when higher and higher doses of epidural narcotics are suggested. Another approach might be to give epidural morphine earlier in labor. The "obstetric" application of the priming principle has been reported to be somewhat successful [35]. When patients were given epidural morphine, 2 mg, at approximately 3-cm cervical dilation followed by bupivacaine, 0.25%, as 5-cm cervical dilation approached (active labor), they achieved better and longer analgesia than patients given bupivacaine in the standard manner (figure 6–9).

Local anesthetics and epidural narcotics

The future of epidural analgesia for labor probably involves the use of more lipid-soluble agents, alone or in combination with local anesthetics. Analgesia has been achieved to some degree with meperidine and fentanyl [36, 37]. However, while the more lipophilic drugs have more rapid onset, their duration of action is short. Epidural meperidine, 100 mg, provided satisfactory pain relief in obstetric patients for only 160.8 ± 90.3 minutes [36]. Would a similar IM dose perhaps be as effective? Certainly a dose level this high strays from the

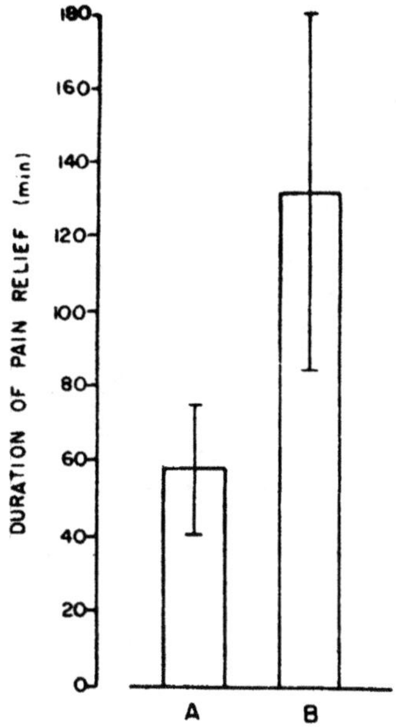

Figure 6–9. The duration in minutes (mean ± SD) of pain relief in groups A and B. Group A was treated with 8 ml epidural 0.25% bupivacaine. Group B was treated with epidural morphine HCL (2 mg in 10 ml of saline) in early labor followed by 8 ml of 0.25% bupivacaine when the patient was in active labor. Pain relief until the next epidural injection was significantly longer in group B than in group A. (Reprinted with permission from Niv D, Valery R, Golan A, Chayan MS. 1986. Augmentation of bupivacaine analgesia in labor by epidural morphine. Obstet Gynecol 67:206–209.)

initial ideal of long-lasting pain relief with very small doses of narcotic. The current trend in this area is the continuous infusion of low-dose lipid-soluble agents like fentanyl or sufentanil in combination with a dilute solution of a local anesthetic and epinephrine. The approach is intriguing and may prove very beneficial.

A second approach of increasing interest is the combination of a local anesthetic with an epidural narcotic [38, 39]. Justins and coworkers demonstrated a faster onset of analgesia in patients given epidural fentanyl (80 μg) and bupivacaine (4 cc of 0.3%), compared with those given IM fentanyl (100 μg) and epidural bupivacaine (4 cc of 0.3%) (figure 6–10) [38]. Similar results have been obtained using sufentanil and bupivacaine [40]. However, with both the local anesthetic and IM combinations, patients' pain scores were very similar within 30 minutes, and the time to first request for further analgesia was not significantly different. A recent study of a similar protocol (epidural fentanyl/bupivacaine combinations) reported *no* difference in the onset of analgesia or the time to maximum analgesia [41]. The authors claimed better

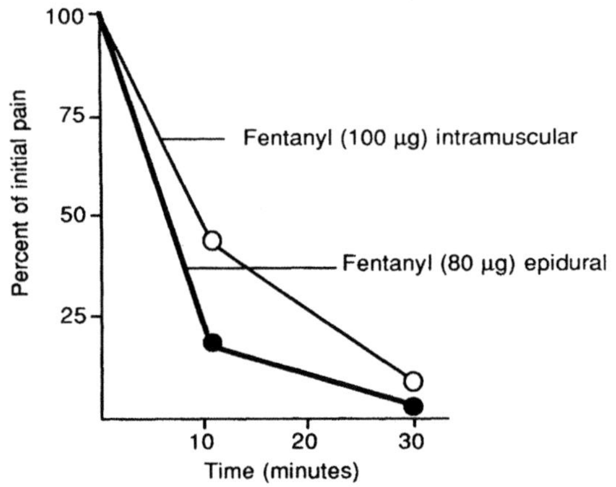

Figure 6–10. Change in pain score after the first epidural injection in the IM fentanyl group (-O-) and in the epidural fentanyl group (-●-). All patients received epidural bupivacaine 12 mg. (Reprinted and adapted with permission of Justins DM, Knott C, Luthman J, Reynolds F. 1983. Epidural versus intramuscular fentanyl. Anaesthesia 38:939–942.)

analgesia was achieved with the combination of drugs, but the visual analogue scale results suggested little clinical significance. Another study using epidural butorphanol and bupivacaine for labor was equally unconvincing, although these investigators suggested a more rapid onset of analgesia [42]. However, the dose of epidural butorphanol (2–3 mg) required to achieve analgesia also caused somnolence in mothers and a sinusoidal fetal heart-rate pattern in apparently 100% of the fetuses of mothers who received 3 mg of epidural butorphanol. The onset of analgesia was more rapid, but all patients obtained similar pain relief 15 minutes after the epidural injection of 0.25% bupivacaine alone or 0.25% bupivacaine with butorphanol. A question arises as to how this technique should be used: Should every top-up dose of a local anesthetic have 2–3 mg of butorphanol?

Yet a third approach is the combined application of epidural lofentanil (1.25 μg) and bupivacaine for labor analgesia, and the application of lofentanil alone (5 μg) for postoperative pain relief. However, the lack of a suitable antagonist for lofentanil makes the use of this drug less appealing [43]. To date, the possible benefits of epidural fentanyl or other lipid-soluble agents for patients in labor have not been clearly demonstrated.

Finally, perhaps the most interesting approach suggested is the use of a continuous infusion (10–16 cc/hr) of very dilute bupivacaine (0.04375%), fentanyl (0.000125%), and epinephrine (1:800,000) (P.C. Youngstrom, personal communications). This technique has been used in over 600 patients with good success. It may be that this combination benefits from three approaches to the neuroaxis, i.e., a local anesthetic and activation of both narcotic and

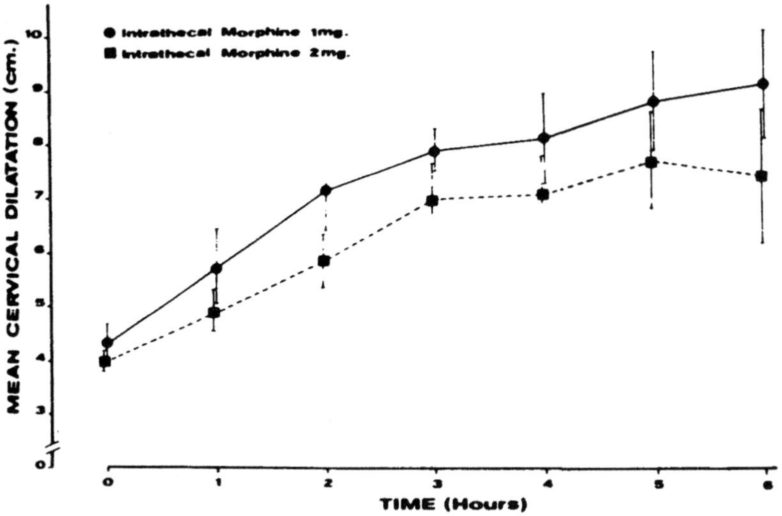

Figure 6–11. The progress of labor and intrathecal morphine cervical dilation versus time. Mean cervical dilation versus time is represented for 7 patients who were given 1 mg of intrathecal morphine and 13 patients given 2 mg. (Reprinted with permission from Baraka A, Noueihid R, Hajj S. 1981. Intrathecal injection of morphine for obstetric analgesia. Anesthesiology 54:136–140.)

adrenergic receptors, and represents the future of epidural narcotics for labor analgesia.

PROGRESS IN LABOR

The effect of traditional regional anesthesia on the progress in labor is an area of research characterized by conflicting data [44]. Intrathecal morphine, 1 mg and 2 mg, reportedly does not affect the progress of labor (figure 6–11) [13]. Similarly, epidural mepeidine, 100 mg, did not affect the progress of labor when compared with 0.25% bupivacaine [36]. However, the administration of epidural fentanyl with bupivacaine may shorten the first stage of labor. In patients receiving this combination, the first stage of labor lasted 430 ± 45 minutes, compared with 602 ± 61 minutes after administration of 0.25% bupivacaine alone [41]. This outcome raised more questions than it answered, and the "striking benefit" the authors suggest in a "significantly shorter first stage of labor" remains to be verified and explained. A continuous infusion (8–10 ml/hr) of bupivacaine, 0.125%, with fentanyl, 1 μg/ml, provided good analgesia without affecting the second stage of labor [45].

THE LIPID-SOLUBLE AGENTS — POSSIBLE USES

In some cases, there may be specific indications for combining a lipid-soluble agent with local anesthetics for analgesia during labor or delivery. Fentanyl,

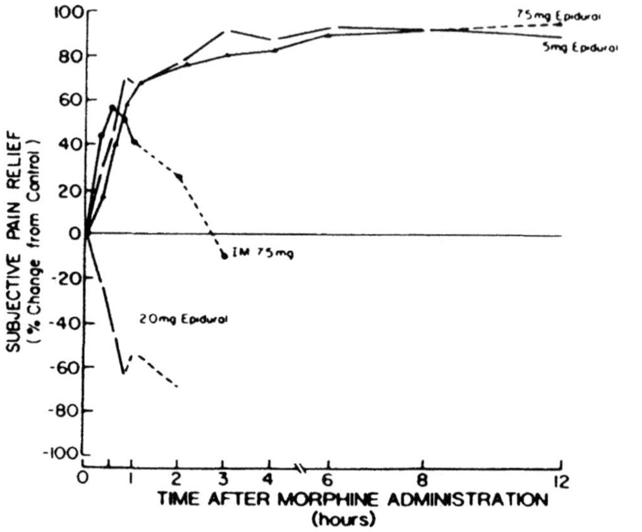

Figure 6–12. Epidural morphine relief of postoperative pain of Caesarean delivery. Note that epidural morphine achieved better pain relief than IM morphine. (Reprinted with permission from Rosen MA, Hughes SC, Shnider SM, Abboud TK, Norton M, Dailey PA, Curtis JD. 1983. Epidural morphine for relief of postoperative pain after Caesarean delivery. Anesth Analg 62: 666–672.)

50–100 μg, added to the epidural regime for low back pain unrelieved by 0.25% bupivacaine, has produced adequate pain relief without further motor blockade — an effect to expect if, instead, the concentration of local anesthetic were increased. This combination would help to maintain the motor tone in the pelvic floor muscles of parturients and perhaps reduce the incidence of forceps delivery. While a single dose of 50–100 μg of epidural fentanyl may be helpful at the start of labor, it would be inappropriate for repeated top-up doses. During Caesarean delivery, the lipid-soluble agents might be helpful when a patient experiences pain upon exteriorization of the uterus in spite of an apparently successful epidural block. Thus, the lipid-soluble agents appear successful for epidural analgesia and may, as a result, become more common in obstetric anesthesia. However, the reader is urged to judge positive reports of their use in obstetric patients carefully, before accepting them into routine practice.

POSTOPERATIVE PAIN: CAESAREAN SECTION

The most rewarding outcome to date has been in the treatment of the postoperative pain of Caesarean delivery. At the University of California, San Francisco (UCSF), we have studied both intrathecal and epidural morphine for labor and delivery, but it is the use of epidural morphine for postoperative pain that has achieved the widest clinical use and is now standard practice. The experience in the obstetric suite has led to the slowly expanding use of this method in our intensive care units and general operating room as well, although the concern for respiratory depression remains a limiting factor. However, epidural morphine simply provides better pain relief in most patients than standard methods. Certainly postoperative pain is often poorly understood and poorly treated by the entire health care team [46]. The earliest work in the Caesarean patients suggested that 100 mg of fentanyl with 8 ml of 0.9% sodium chloride administered via an epidural catheter could provide good postoperative pain relief [47]. Rosen and coworkers at UCSF performed a dose–response study of postoperative pain relief following Caesarean section, in which they compared epidural morphine, 2 mg, 5 mg, and 7.5 mg, with IM morphine, 7.5 mg, in patients who had received epidural anesthesia [48]. The lower dose was chosen to confirm the findings of Behar et al. However, 2 mg proved ineffective in these patients, while the two higher doses were equally satisfactory (figure 6–12). The duration of analgesia was 29 hours 12 minutes (± 3.6 hours) with the 5-mg dose of epidural morphine.

We now use preservative-free epidural morphine [Duramorph P.F., Elkins-Sinn], 5 mg, as part of our routine postoperative regime following Caesarean delivery under regional anesthesia [49]. Others have confirmed this dose range although this author has suggested using 3.5–4.0 mg of morphine, leaving the catheter in, and titrating further narcotic to effect if more pain relief is required [50–53]. We most often place the dose through the epidural catheter after the umbilical cord is clamped and then remove the catheter at the end of surgery. Certainly 2.0 mg of morphine is ineffective [54–56]. In another dose–response study, Bromage and coworkers administered various narcotics in incremental doses until satisfactory analgesia was achieved [57]. In the group given epidural morphine (a mixed group of surgical patients), 10.3 mg (± 2.5 SD) was required following upper abdominal surgery and 7.5 mg (± 2.1 SD) following lower abdominal surgery. Our dose for lower abdominal surgery (Caesarean section) is slightly less, and a similar dose range was suggested by Stenseth et al. after their experience with more than 1000 general surgical patients [58].

Both the surgical procedure and the individual's response to pain potentially alter the dose requirements. Allen et al. suggested epidural morphine, 5 mg, for postoperative pain relief after knee surgery and vascular surgery [59]. However, their vascular surgical group achieved greater duration of pain relief (24 hours versus 16.6 hours), indicating that different surgical procedures can alter epidural narcotic requirements (figure 6–13). Thus, the "recipe" for Caesarean delivery patients at UCSF cannot necessarily be used in other groups of patients with the same effect, but with titration of the dose, pain relief can be achieved. Individuals within a specific surgical group also vary in their response to pain and in the dose required to relieve pain.

At UCSF, we recently reviewed the first 1000 patients given epidural morphine, 5 mg, after Caesarean delivery and found that 85% achieved good

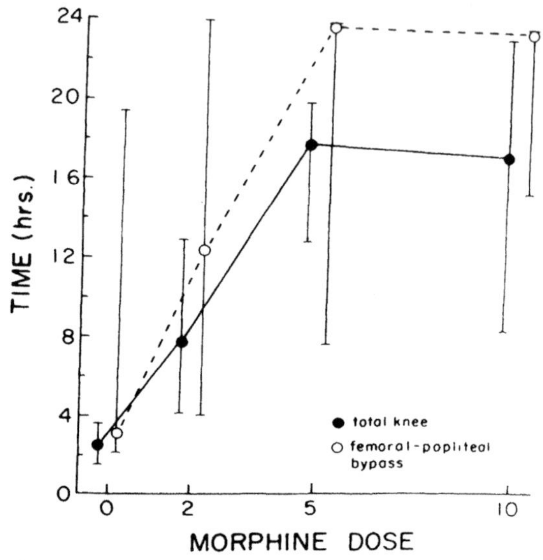

Figure 6–13. Time to first requested parenteral medication after administration of study drug (median ± quartile), epidural morphine. Patients had received epidural anesthesia with bupivacaine 0.5% for their surgical procedure. There is a significant relationship between time and dose in both treatment groups ($p < 0.003$) and a significant difference between the two control groups ($p < 0.05$). (Reprinted with permission From Allen PD, Walman T, Concepcion M, Sheskey M, Patterson MK, Cullen D, Covino BF. 1986. Epidural morphine provides postoperative pain relief in peripheral vascular and orthopedic surgical patients: A dose–response study. Anesth Analg 65:165–170.)

to excellent analgesia with a mean duration of 23 ± 0.4 hours [60]. For the 20% who obtained less than 12 hours of analgesia, leaving the epidural catheter in and adding further narcotics as required would solve this problem. Considering the individual response to pain therapy, 16% of patients did not request further analgesics (oral or parenteral) during their hospital stay and 44% required only oral analgesics. Pruritus was the most common side effect, occurring in 61% of the patients. Although only 4% described their pruritus as severe, 29% requested and received treatment. Nausea occurred in 20% of patients who were treated variably with low-dose naloxone (.1–.2 mg), droperidol (0.625–1.25 mg IV), or metoclopramide (10 mg IV). A similar incidence of nausea might be expected after IM morphine for abdominal surgery. None of the 96 patients who received droperidol for nausea experienced respiratory depression, a previously reported potential side effect [61]. While one must always consider the possible synergistic actions of any IV or IM medication administered to a patient who has received intraspinal narcotics, pain, nausea, and vomiting can and must be treated. Our review revealed only four cases of respiratory depression, indicated by patients having a respiratory rate of 10 or lower [60]. Two of these patients were observed closely and did not require further treatment. The third patient received IV naloxone to treat a respiratory rate of nine, but an arterial blood gas sample taken as the patient was given naloxone revealed normal blood gas values, indicating that the patient was not in respiratory distress. The fourth patient in this group showed a slow but progressive decrease in the respiratory rate from 20 breaths/min to 4–6 breaths/min and alarming arterial blood gas values (pH = 7.08, pCO_2 = 76, pO_2 = 40, and BE = −6). The arterial sample was drawn as naloxone and oxygen were being given. The patient responded promptly to naloxone (0.1 mg) and oxygen administered by mask. It would appear to be significant that the decline in respiratory rate was gradual. While the patient's distress was noted by our monitoring system and tracked by the nursing staff, naloxone could have been administered earlier in the course of events. Thus, our standing orders have been changed to allow the nursing staff freedom in administering naloxone.

Our data suggest that the incidence of potentially life-threatening respiratory depression in the UCSF population may be as low as 0.1%. This agrees with data from Rawal et al., who suggest a 0.09% incidence of respiratory depression after epidural morphine (N = 14,000) [62]. The Rawal group included general surgery, chronic pain, and trauma patients. While there are few good data of which we are aware on the incidence of respiratory depression in postoperative patients given routine intramuscular narcotics, the suggested rate of life-threatening respiratory depression is 0.9% [63]. Despite the lower risk associated with intraspinal narcotics, careful monitoring is necessary and resuscitative treatment must be immediately available. Once a patient has demonstrated sedation or respiratory depression, vigilant monitoring is required. A naloxone drip of 5–10 μg/kg may be indicated in such patients to prevent further respiratory depression. Smaller doses of naloxone are probably inappropriate and ineffective [64].

We monitor our patients on the routine obstetric ward, but also ensure careful nursing and good communication among all individuals caring for the patient. We follow a specific monitoring protocol (table 6–2). While some authors have suggested apnea monitors, end-tidal CO_2 monitors, intensive care monitoring, "Victorian wards," or transcutaneous O_2 or CO_2 monitoring, we have been successful with excellent nursing and a stringent monitoring protocol. It is possible, however, that the obstetric patient is different from the routine surgical patient with respect to respiratory drive, and this subject is being investigated. Stenseth et al. have reported a low incidence of respiratory depression in a large general surgical population receiving epidural anesthesia [58]. However, older patients having pulmonary disease might be at greater risk for respiratory depression [65]. Certainly, obstetric patients are younger, usually have minimal or no pulmonary disease, and have elevated levels of progesterone, the effects of which cannot be discounted. However, it is important that patients be in an area in which resuscitative equipment, oxygen, naloxone, and other resuscitative drugs are immediately available.

Table 6–2. Suggested postoperative intraspinal orders

1. The patient has received the following:
   Morphine ______ mg or______________
   Route: Epidural ______ Intrathecal ______
   Date ______________ Time ____________
2. Bed and Kardex to be labeled "Intraspinal Narcotic Patient."
3. Naloxone (naloxone) ampule (1 ml, 0.4 mg) and syringe must be readily available at the nursing station.
4. Oxygen flow meter with nipple adapter and self-inflating bag with mask must be immediately accessible, either at nursing station or at patient's bedside.
5. No PO, IM, IV, or SQ narcotics are to be given for 24 hours, except by order of or after consultation with an anesthesiologist: beeper #______.
6. Check and record respiratory rate q 30 min for 12 hrs, then q 1 hr until 24 hrs after intraspinal narcotic administration.
7. Call anesthesiologist (beeper #______) and house officer if:
   a) Respiratory rate is below 11,
   b) Evidence of airway obstruction,
   c) Change in respiratory pattern,
   d) Decreased respiratory effort, or
   e) Pin-point pupils or patient is very drowsy.
8. If respiratory rate is $<$ 8/min or patient is in respiratory distress, house officer or nurse may administer Narcan 0.2 mg IV (0.5 ml), and repeat as necessary.
9. Keep open IV infusion or heparin lock.
10. Treatment of nausea, vomiting, pruritus interfering with normal activity, or urinary retention:
    a) Narcan 0.1 mg (0.25 mg) q 15 min $\times$ 3, PRN IV bolus; PRN Q 4–6^0
    b) If no relief by 45 min, start Narcan infusion at 0.2 mg/hr:
       (1.6 mg or 4.0 ml Narcan in 1,000 ml at 125 ml/hr or
       0.8 mg or 2.0 ml Narcan in 500 ml at 125 ml/hr or
       0.4 mg or 1.0 ml Narcan in 250 ml at 125 ml/hr)
    c) If symptoms are not improved by 60 min of infusion, increase rate to 0.4 mg/hr (by adding more Narcan to IV fluids).
    d) Pitoicin and Narcan are compatible and can be mixed together.
    e) Discontinue Narcan infusion after 3 hr. If pruritus returns, restart Narcan infusion for an additional 3 hr.
    f) If surgical pain returns, stop infusion and call anesthesia resident.
    g) Metoclopramide 10 mg IV q 2 hr for nausea not relieved by Narcan.
11. Call anesthesiologist (beeper #______) if patient complains of incomplete pain relief or severe itching, urinary retention, excessive nausea, or vomiting not improved by treatment with Narcan.
12. Activity: As tolerate.

Particular attention should be paid to patients' vital signs when they receive additional narcotics or sedative drugs to supplement analgesia or a waning epidural dose. The combined effect of a small amount of residual epidural narcotic in the CSF with a systemic plasma concentration of narcotic from an IM or IV injection could be catastrophic. Although this has not occurred in our practice, we consider it a potential risk. When the epidural narcotic and analgesia wanes and additional medication is first requested, we usually give a healthy dose of narcotic and observe for the possible combined effect. After that, routine postoperative pain orders can be implemented.

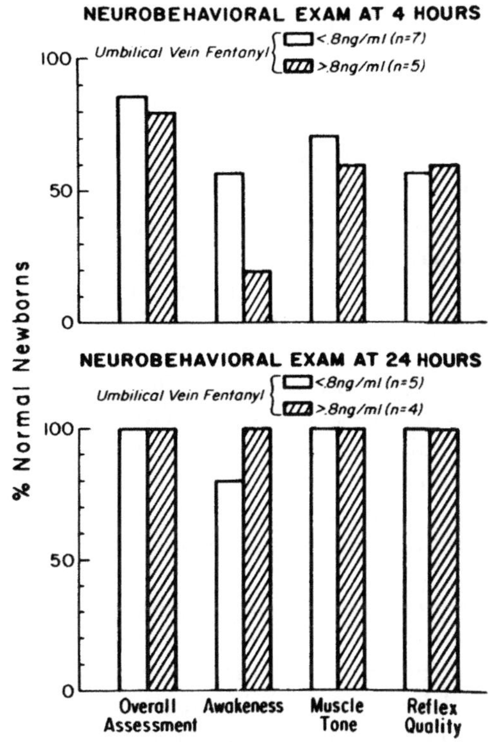

Figure 6–14. Neurobehavioral examination at 4 hours (top) and 24 hours (bottom) comparing newborns with umbilical cord fentanyl concentrations less than and more than 0.8 ng/ml at delivery. the mothers had received 1 mg/kg of IV fentanyl just before Caesarean section. The percentage of newborns having normal scores is shown for each of four categories: overall assessment, awakeness, muscle tone, and reflex quality. Newborns having high cord concentrations of fentanyl received low scores for awakeness at 4 hours. Those with lower cord fentanyl concentrations were similar to the control group at 4 hours. (Reprinted with permission from Eisele JH, Wright R, Rogge P. 1982. Newborn and maternal fentanyl levels at Caesarean section. Anesth Analg 61:179.)

NEONATAL EFFECTS

Extensive investigation has documented the safe use of intrathecal (0.5–2 mg) and epidural morphine sulfate (2–7.5 mg) [11–14]. Intrathecal morphine was found to produce analgesia in the gravid rat and has no effect upon parturition [66]. Hughes and coworkers noted high Apgar and Neurological and Adaptive Capacity scores, and normal values for umbilical arterial and venous blood gas tensions in newborns delivered of mothers given 2 mg, 5 mg, and 7.5 mg of epidural morphine [12]. Because the doses administered to the mothers were small, this outcome is not surprising. However, the rapid placental transfer of epidural narcotics has been documented, and if repeated doses of epidural narcotics are given or if significant amounts of narcotics are continuously infused, a depressed infant could result. In some cases, a plasma concentration as low as 1 ng/ml may depress a newborn; this concentration may be reached when 1 μg/kg of drug is administered epidurally or intravenously, although clinical reports vary. This fentanyl dose is under investigation as a possible additive to 2% epidural lidocaine for Caesarean section, for example, and should probably not be used if there is any evidence of a compromised neonate. At UCSF, we are currently evaluating the neonatal effects of such an approach. As discussed earlier, fentanyl and other lipid-soluble narcotics are now being considered as epidural agents for labor in combination with a local anesthetic. Fentanyl is said to potentiate epidural bupivacaine 0.25%, the most common local anesthetic agent used during labor. If the dosage applied is carefully limited, fentanyl should have little effect on the newborn although it does cross the placenta rapidly and has been shown to affect neurobehavioral outcome, especially awakeness (figure 6–14) at four hours postpartum [9]. However, all neonatal effects had cleared at 24 hours, and it has been suggested that fentanyl is a useful adjuvant for either regional or general anesthesia for Caesarean delivery, and in limited doses may be an appropriate epidural agent [7].

There is an increasing interest in giving a continuous infusion of naloxone to decrease the side effects of intraspinal narcotics. A continuous IV infusion of naloxone (0.4–0.6 mg/hr) in parturients who had received intrathecal morphine (0.5–1 mg) for labor decreased the incidence of pruritus (35% with IV saline versus 9% with IV naloxone) and had no effect upon the newborn [67]. The plasma concentration of naloxone (1.92 ± 0.28 ng/ml) in the umbilical venous blood was low. Dailey and coworkers also noted no difference between β-endorphin levels in newborns whose mothers were given IV naloxone and those whose mothers had received IV saline (control group). The Dailey study confirmed that low-dose intrathecal morphine or IV naloxone during labor had no effect on the newborn. However, the continuous infusion of IV naloxone tended to shorten the duration of maternal analgesia achieved with intrathecal morphine. Rawal et al. have demonstrated a 25% decrease in postoperative pain relief provided by epidural morphine when a continuous infusion of naloxone was given [68]. This would probably not be a problem in the parturient receiving intraspinal narcotics and IV naloxone, unless a very long labor resulted. While naloxone administered to the hypoxic fetus has been reported to increase hypoxic brain damage, current data are inconclusive [69, 70]. The American Academy of Pediatrics recommends repeated IV bolus administration of 10 μg/kg of naloxone to the infant suspected of narcotization, and this has been successful [71]. This dose is well above that likely to be recommended for IV administration of naloxone to a parturient who has received intraspinal narcotics.

While the use of intraspinal narcotics is a changing area of research and clinical investigation, the work to date confirms one of the initial hypotheses of intraspinal narcotics: long-lasting analgesia can be provided for the parturient using small doses of intraspinal narcotics that have minimal effect on the newborn. The reader is urged, however, to examine new recipes for labor analagesia with the safety of the newborn clearly in mind.

CONCLUSIONS

The use of intraspinal narcotics for labor and delivery is getting a fresh look. Intrathecal morphine is clearly effective, but the well-known side effects, including postdural puncture headache, are not to be overlooked. Combined epidural application of more lipid-soluble narcotics, a local anesthetic, and an adrenergic agent is of great interest, but hard data demonstrating its effectiveness and benefit are slow to accumulate. Thus, modulation of the neuroaxis to achieve solid analgesia for labor without the use of local anesthetic remains only a tantalizing possibility, but an area of great interest and research activity.

The benefits of intraspinal narcotics to the Caesarean delivery patient are evident. Better pain relief is achieved with epidural morphine (5 mg) than with the usual IM approach or patient-controlled analgesia [72]. This alone should be enough reason to use this technique. There are growing claims of a shorter hospital stay, better pulmonary function in the postoperative period, and earlier ambulation after surgery, but these have yet to be conclusively demonstrated and to achieve widespread acceptance [73]. However, the benefits of intraspinal narcotics for the treatment of postoperative pain in the obstetric patient appear to be great and the risks minimal.

REFERENCES

1. Hughes SC. 1987. Intraspinal opiates in obstetrics. In Shnider SM, Levinson G, (eds): Anesthesia for Obstetrics, 2nd ed. Philadelphia: Williams and Wilkins, chapter 10.
2. Wang JK, Nauss LA, Thomas JE. 1979. Pain relief by intrathecally applied morphine in man. Anesthesiology 50:149–151.
3. Behar M, Magora F, Olshwang D, Davidson JT. 1979. Epidural morphine in treatment of pain. Lancet i:527–528.
4. Downes JJ, Kemp RA, Lambersen CJ. 1967. The magnitude and duration of respiratory depression due to fentanyl and meperidine in man. J Pharmacol Exp Ther 158:416–420.
5. Forrest WH, Bellville JW. 1968. Respiratory effects of alphaprodine in man. Obstet Gynecol 31:61–68.
6. Fuller JD, Crombleholme WR. 1987 Respiratory arrest and prolonged respiratory depression after one low, subcutaneous dose of alphaprodine for obstetric analgesia. J Reprod Med 32:149–151.
7. Levinson G, Shnider SM. 1987. Systemic medication for labor and delivery. In Shnider SM, Levinson G (eds): Anesthesia for Obstetrics, 2nd ed. Philadelphia: Williams and Wilkins, chapter 8.
8. Nybell-Lindahl G, Carlsson C, Ingemarsson I, Westgren M, Paalzow L. 1981. Maternal and fetal concentrations of morphine after epidural administration during labor. Am J Obstet Gynecol 139:20–21.
9. Eisele JH. 1984. The use of short-acting narcotics is obstetric anesthesia and the effects on the newborn. In Estafanous FG (ed): Opioids in Anesthesia. Boston: Butterworth Publishers, chapter 8.
10. Ainslie FG, Eisele JH, Corkill G. 1979. Fentanyl concentrations in brain and the serum during respiratory acid-base changes in the dog. Anesthesiology 51:295–297.
11. Scott PV, Bowen FE, Cartwright P, Rao BCM, Deeley D, Wotherspoon HG, Sumrein IMA.

1980. Intrathecal morphine as sole analgesic during labour. Br J Med 281:351–353.
12. Hughes SC, Rosen MA, Shnider SM, Abboud TK, Stefani SJ, Morton M. 1984. Maternal and neonatal effects of epidural morphine for labor and delivery. Anesth Analg 63:319–324.
13. Baraka A, Noueihid R, Hajj S. 1981. Intrathecal injection of morphine for obstetric analgesia. Anesthesiology 54:136–140.
14. Abboud TK, Shnider SM, Dailey PA, Raya JA, Sarkis F, Grobler NM, Sadri S, Khoo SS, DeSousa B, Baysinger CL, Miller F. 1984. Intrathecal administration of hyperbaric morphine for the relief of pain in labour. Br J Anaesth 56:1351–1360.
15. Nordberg G, Hedner T, Mellstrand T, Dahlström B. 1984. Pharmacokinetic aspects of intrathecal morphine analgesia. Anesthesiology 60:448–454.
16. Glass PSA, Biagi B, Sischy S, Camporesi E. 1985. Analgesic action of very low dose intrathecal morphine (0.1 mg) as compared to high doses (0.2–0.4 mg). Anesthesiology 63:A236.
17. Cunningham AJ, McKenna JA, Skene DS. 1983. Single injection spinal anesthesia with tetracaine and morphine for transurethral prostatectomy. Anesth Analg 62:255.
18. Brizgys RV, Shnider SM. 1984. Hyperbaric intrathecal morphine analgesia during labor in a patient with Wolff–Parkinson–White Syndrome. Obstet Gynecol 64:445–465.
19. Hyde NH, Horison DM. 1986. Intrathecal morphine in a parturient with cystic fibrosis. Anesth Analg 65:1357–1358.
20. Milne B, Cervenko FW, Thamandas K, Sutak M. 1985. Intrathecal clonidine: Analgesia and effect on opiate withdrawal in the rat. Anesthesiology 62:34–38.
21. Reddy SV, Laderut L, Yaksh TL. 1980. Spinal pharmacology of adrenergic agonist-mediated antinociception. J Pharmacol Exp Ther 213:525–533.
22. Eisenach JC, Rose JC, Dewan DM. 1986. Epidural clonidine antinociception in sheep. Anesthesiology 65:A192.
23. Abouleish EI. 1986. Epinephrine improves the quality of spinal anesthesia of bupivacaine. Anesthesiology 65:A375.
24. Bion JF. 1984. Intrathecal ketamine for war surgery. A preliminary study under field conditions. Anaesthesia 39:1023–1028.
25. Ahuja BR. 1983. Analgesic effect of intrathecal ketamine in rats. Br J Anaesth 55:991–995.
26. Brock-Utne JG, Mankowitz E, Kalhichurum S, Downing JW. 1982. Effects of intrathecal saline and ketamine with and without preservative on the spinal nerve roots of monkeys. S Afr Med J 61:360–361.
27. Mirelles FS, Lopez-Soriano F, Perez D, Lopez-Rodriguez F, Puig MM. 1986. Subarachnoid administration of calcitonin produces postoperative analgesia. Anesthesiology 65:A199.
28. Börner U, Müller H, Stoganov M, Hempelmann G. 1980. Epidurale opiate analgesie, Gewebe-und liquor vertäglich keit der opiate. Anaesthesist 29:570–571.
29. Hussemeyer RP, O'Connor MC, Davenport HT. 1980. Failure of epidural morphine to relieve pain in labour. Anaesthesia 35:161–163.
30. Writer WDR, James FM III, Wheeler AS. 1981. Double-blind comparison of morphine and bupivacaine for continuous epidural analgesia in labor. Anesthesiology 54:215–219.
31. Booker PD, Wilkes RG, Bryson THL, Beddard J. 1980. Obstetric pain relief using epidural morphine. Anaesthesia 35:377–379.
32. Crawford JS. 1981. Forum experiences with epidural morphine in obstetrics. Anaesthesia 36:207–209.
33. Von Hartung H-J, Wiest W, Klose R, Bauknecht H, Hettenbach A. 1980. Epidurale morphine-injektion zur schmerzbekämpfung in her geburtshilfe. Fortschr Med 98:500.
34. Dick W, Traub E, Moller RM. 1982. Epidural morphine in obstetric anesthesia. Obstet Anesth Digest 2(1):29–31.
35. Niv D, Volery R, Golan A, Chayen MS. 1986. Augmentation of bupivacaine analgesia in labor by epidural morphine. Obstet Gynecol 67:206–209.
36. Baraka A, Maktabi M, Noueihid R. 1982. Epidural meperidine–bupivacaine for obstetric analgesia. Anesth Analg 61:652–656.
37. Nalda MA, Campo F, Burzaco I. 1982. Obstetric analgesia with fentanyl–bupivacaine by the extradural route. Br J Anaesth 54:250P.
38. Justins DM, Knott C, Luthman J, Reynolds F. 1983. Epidural versus intramuscular fentanyl. Anaesthesia 38:937–942.
39. Youngstrom P, Eastwood D, Patel H, Bhatia R, Cowen R, Sutheiner C. 1984. Epidural

fentanyl and bupivacaine in labor: A double-blind study. Anesthesiology 61:A414.
40. Phillips G. 1987. Epidural sufentanil in labor. Anesth Analg 66:S140.
41. Cohen SE, Tan S, Albright GA, Halpern J. 1986. Epidural fentanyl/bupivacaine combinations for labor analgesia: Effect of varying dosages. Anesthesiology 65:A368.
42. Naulty JS, Malinow A, Hunt CO, Hausheer J, Datta S, Lema MJ, Ostheimer GW. 1986. Epidural butorphanol–bupivacaine for analgesia during labor and delivery. Anesthesiology 65:A369.
43. Van Steenberge A. 1985. Epidural lofentanil for pain relief in labor. Anesthezie Intenzivmedizin 31:394–397.
44. DeVore JS, Eisler EA. 1987. Effects of anesthesia on uterine activity and labor. In Shnider SM, Levinson G, (eds): Anesthesia for Obstetrics, 2nd ed. Philadelphia: Williams and Wilkins, chapter 4.
45. Bochenet KJ, Iovan SN, Brouwn EM. 1987. Continuous infusion epidural 0.12% bupivacaine/fentanyl and the second stage of labor. Anesth Analg S15.
46. Weis O, Sriwatanakul K, Alloza JL, Weintraub M, Lasagna L. 1983. Attitudes of patients, house staff, and nurses toward postoperative analgesic care. Anesth Analg 62:70–74.
47. Wolfe MJ, Nicholas ADG. 1979. Selective epidural analagesia. Lancet i:150–151.
48. Rosen MA, Hughes SC, Shnider SM, Abboud TK, Norton M, Dailey PA, Curtis JD. 1983. Epidural morphine for relief of postoperative pain after Cesarean delivery. Anesth Analg 62:666–672.
49. Kotelko DM, Dailey PA, Shnider SM, Rosen MA, Hughes SC, Brizgys RV. 1984. Epidural morphine analgesia after Cesarean delivery. Obstet Gynecol 63:409–413.
50. Youngstrom PC, Cowan RI, Suthheimer C, Eastwood DW, Yu JCM. 1982. Pain relief and plasma concentrations from epidural and intramuscular morphine in post-Cesarean patients. Anesthesiology 57:404–409.
51. Coombs DW, Danielson DR, Pageau MG, Rippe E. 1982. Epidurally administered morphine for postcesarean analgesia. Surg Gynecol Obstet 154:385–388.
52. Carmichael FJ, Rolbin SH, Hew EM. 1982. Epidural morphine for analgesia after Cesarean section. Can Anaesth Soc J 29:359–363.
53. Binsted RJ. 1983. Epidural morphine after Cesarean section. Anaesth Intensive Care 11:130–134.
54. Chayen MS, Rudick V, Borvine A. 1980. Pain control with epidural injection of morphine. Anesthesiology 53:338–339.
55. Rawal N, Sjöstrand U, Dahlström B. 1981. Postoperative pain relief by epidural morphine. Anesth Analg 60:726–731.
56. Yu CM, Youngstrom PC, Cowan RI, Spagnuolo SET. 1980. Postcesarean epidural morphine: Double-blind study. Anesthesiology 53S:216.
57. Bromage PR, Camporesi E, Chestnut D. 1980. Epidural narcotics for postoperative analgesia. Anesth Analg 59:473–480.
58. Stenseth R, Sellevold O, Brievik H. 1985. Epidural morphine for postoperative pain: Experience with 1085 patients. Acta Anaesthesiol Scand 29:148–156.
59. Allen PD, Walman T, Concepcion M, Sheskey M, Patterson MK, Cullen D, Covino BF. 1986. Epidural morphine provides postoperative pain relief in peripheral vascular and orthopedic surgical patients: A dose–response study. Anesth Analg 65:165–170.
60. Leicht CH, Hughes SC, Dailey PA, Shnider SM, Rosen MA. 1986. Epidural morphine sulfate for analgesia after Cesarean section: A postoperative report of 1000 patients. Anesthesiology 65:A366.
61. Cohen SE, Rothblatt AJ, Albright GA. 1983. Early respiratory depression with epidural narcotic and intravenous droperidol. Anesthesiology 59:559–560.
62. Rawal N, Arnér S, Gustafsson LL, Allvin R. 1987. Present state of epidural and intrathecal opiate analgesia — A nationwide follow-up survey in Sweden. Br J Anaesth 59:791–799.
63. Miller RR, Greenblatt DJ. 1976. Drug effects in hospitalized patients. Experiences of the Boston collaborative drug surveillance program 1966–1975. Wiley Biomedical, p. 151.
64. Ramanathan S, Horn R, Parker F, Turndorf H. 1986. Naloxone infusion is ineffective in preventing the side-effects of epidural morphine in post-Cesarean section patients. Anesthesiology 65:A367.
65. Gustafsson LL, Schildt B, Jacobsen K. 1982. Adverse effects of extradural and intrathecal opiates: Report of a nationwide survey in Sweden. Br J Anaesth 54:479–486.

66. Yaksh TL, Wilson PR, Kaiko RF, Inturrisi CE. 1979. Analgesia produced by a spinal action of morphine and effects upon parturition in the rat. Anesthesiology 51:386–392.
67. Dailey PA, Brookshire GL, Shnider SM, Abboud TK, Kotelko DM, Noueihid R, Thigpen JW, Khoo SS, Raya JA, Foutz SE, Brizgys RV, Goebelsman U, Lo MW. 1984. Naloxone decreases side effects after intrathecal morphine for labor. Anesth Analg 64:658–666.
68. Rawal N, Schött U, Dahlström B, Inturrisi CE, Tandon B, Sjöstrand U, Wennhager M. 1986. Influence of naloxone infusion on analgesia and respiratory depression following epidural morphine. Anesthesiology 64:194–201.
69. Young RSK, Hesert TR, Pritchard GA, Yagel SK. 1984. Naloxone exacerbates hypoxic–ischemic brain injury in the neonatal rat. Am J Obstet Gynecol 50:52–56.
70. La Bamma EF, Itskovitz J, Rudolph AM. 1982. Effects of naloxone on fetal circulatory responses to hypoxemia. Am J Obstet Gynecol 143:933.
71. Segal S, Anyan WR Jr, Hill RM, Kauffman RE, Mofenson H, Pruitt AW, Shniefield HR, Singer HAS, Weinberger MM. 1980. Committee on drugs. Naloxone use in newborns. Pediatrics 65:667–669.
72. Harrison DM, Sinatra RS, Morgese L, Chung JH, Mandel ALZ. 1986. Epidural and patient controlled analgesia for post-Cesarean section pain relief. Anesthesiology 65:A364.
73. Rawal N, Sjöstrand U, Christoffersson E, Dahlström B, Arvill A, Rydman H. 1984. Comparison of intramuscular and epidural morphine for postoperative analgesia in the grossly obese: Influence on postoperative ambulation and pulmonary function. Anesth Analg 63:583–592.

7. DELIVERY SYSTEMS FOR CHRONIC SPINAL ANALGESIA

DENNIS W. COOMBS

A substantial and growing technology is available to the clinician contemplating spinal narcotic therapy. Indeed, the flexibility of current technology in this area lends spinal narcotic therapy some of its principal advantages, i.e., reversibility and interchangeability. By comparison with neurolytic blockade, pain control with spinal analgesics may be achieved with a variety of interchangeable or coadministered agents with variable duration but reversible antinociceptive action. The choice of a spinal delivery system is ultimately dictated by individual patient need. However, awareness of the potential alternatives is necessary in order to appreciate the best choice for a given patient and to troubleshoot when malfunction occurs.

The three basic types of delivery systems have been reviewed elsewhere recently [1, 2]. The three options include 1) a percutaneously implanted spinal catheter (usually epidural in location) with or without subcutaneous tunnelling, 2) subcutaneously implanted injection ports, and 3) implanted infusion reservoirs. The technical details of implantation of spinal delivery systems have been covered elsewhere, and only important practical issues that relate particularly to specific systems will be stressed [3–6].

CHRONIC SPINAL ANALGESIC DELIVERY SYSTEMS

A variety of catheter types and materials have been employed for chronic spinal analgesic delivery, including nylon, silicone, polyamide, teflon, and perhaps others. Little chronic study has been undertaken to identify the

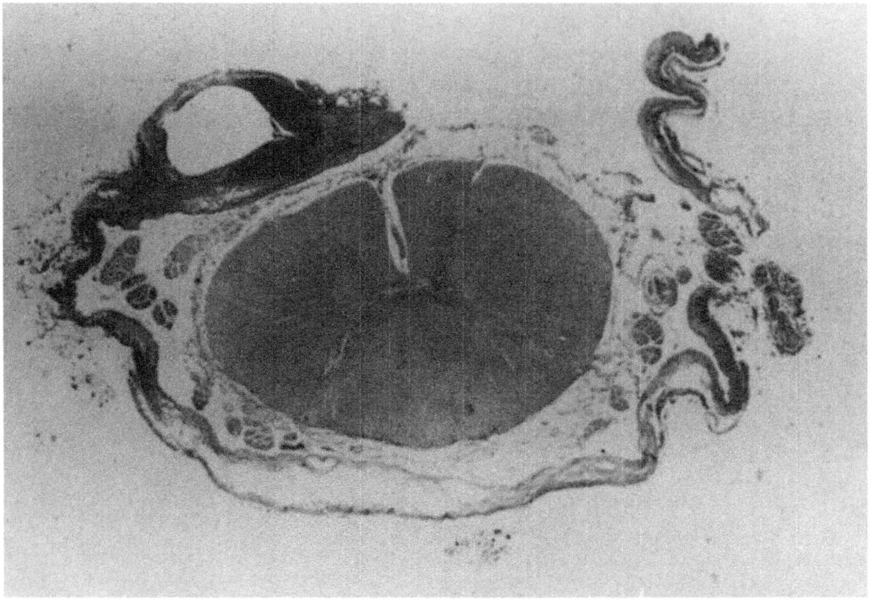

Figure 7–1. Low-power cross section of lumbar spinal cord, leptomeninges, and epidural catheter tract from a patient with indwelling epidural silicone catheter in place for six months of continuous epidural morphine infusion. Note thickened dura and pericatheter fibrosis with adjacent area of necrosis.

reactivity of such systems to leptomeninges [7]. Our chronic spinal implants in dog, sheep, and man have revealed that some degree of leptomeningeal fibrosis occurs [7, 8]. Figure 7–1 is a low-power photomicrograph of the spinal cord and leptomeninges in a cancer patient who died after six months of epidural morphine therapy. The spinal cord is normal; however, a substantially thickened dura surrounds the silicone epidural catheter with even some focal necrosis near the catheter. Such reactivity may potentially lead to painful injection, catheter obstruction, decreased dural penetration of drug, local spinal cord compression, and perhaps generalized arachnoiditis [7–10]. Fortunately, such reactions have been rarely reported at postmortem in chronically treated patients. Further research is still needed to specifically identify the best catheter material for chronic use.

Several points regarding spinal catheter implantation will be emphasized. First, in this author's opinion, a softer, flexible catheter material is preferable, despite being slightly more difficult to implant. Silicone is easiest to anchor against inadvertent removal without the risk of kink or break associated with less flexible materials, i.e., teflon. This author prefers to anchor percutaneous catheters to the supraspinous ligament, and if tunnelled, also to the skin.

Obviously, the latter procedure requires a small incision over the desired spinal interspace. Additionally, silicone is an approved chronic implantable conduit for neurosurgical indications, i.e., lumbar peritoneal shunts, with obvious medicolegal consequences in the event of a neurological injury during chronic spinal drug therapy, i.e., paresis or arachnoiditis.

Implantation of a chronic spinal catheter deserves attention to aseptic detail and care to prevent neurological complications. The skin over the implantation areas should be free of decubitis, infection, or irritation. Prophylactic antibiotic coverage is especially recommended for implanted systems. Ideally, coagulation studies should be within normal limits. Fluoroscopic control is useful to identify catheter position and to rule out inadvertent cannulation of veins, subdural space, or intrathecal space (if epidural placement was intended).

Several considerations make a percutaneous epidural catheter the commonest choice among delivery systems. In increasing order of importance, the low expense to the patient, short duration of anticipated survival, and good support systems to provide help during home care of the patient all weight one's judgment in favor of a percutaneous system. The need to use local anesthetic for pain control necessitates two clinical decisions: 1) an epidural rather than intrathecal catheter, and 2) placement of the catheter close to the dermatomal level associated with the origin of the pain. The use of local anesthetic may be necessary to treat neurogenic pain resistant to spinal narcotic, to treat reflex-sympathetic dystrophy, or to provide pain relief while spinal narcotic is being withdrawn. No definite contraindication exists against extended use of percutaneous spinal catheters, though this may preclude chronic intrathecal drug administration due to risk of meningitis [11]. Several large series have been reported indicating that extended therapy is possible, although with some increased risk of both local infection and accidental catheter dislodgement. In Andersen's series of over 600 cases treated with chronic epidural morphine, an average of two catheters per patient was required, but the range was from one to six per patient [12]. Thus it is essential to have ready availability of trained personnel to replace dislodged, kinked, or obstructed catheters, or when pain on injection requires relocation of the catheter. These series reported by Zenz et al. and Andersen and colleagues suggest that the risk of infection is between 5% and 10%, with rare cases of meningitis also being reported [11, 12].

Figure 7–2 shows a patient with a tunnelled epidural catheter in place. No clear evidence exists that tunnelling will reduce the incidence of infection. However, the experience with hyperalimentation catheters suggests that this may be so. DuPenn and colleagues have recently reported a modified silicone epidural catheter with a Broviac-type cuff for implantation [13]. The initial series suggests reasonable reliability and infection rates. There remain occasional cases of obstruction and pain on injection.

Percutaneous systems may be disadvantagous, especially when support per-

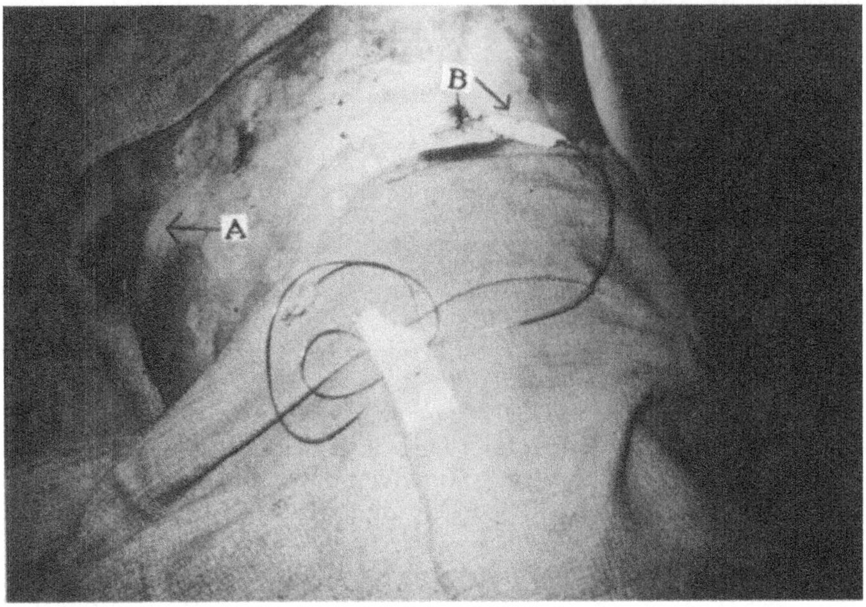

Figure 7–2. Percutaneously tunnelled thoracic epidural catheter (polyamide, Burron, Inc., Melsungen, W. Germany) for treatment of lung cancer-associated chest wall pain.
Arrow A: Catheter placement incision in the spine.
Arrow B: Skin-anchoring suture is tied to mole skin that has been wrapped around the catheter. Mole skin helps prevent anchoring suture from compression occlusion of the catheter.

sonnel for repeated injections are not readily available. Table 7–1 lists some of the factors that make other alternatives desirable or necessary. Especially notable are rare cases of sensitivity to the sedative effects of narcotics, particularly in the elderly. Totally implanted systems require only a slight modification from a percutaneously tunnelled system, namely creation of a subcutaneous pocket for the delivery reservoir. Implanted catheter ports may be located either intrathecally or epidurally. Obviously, if local anesthetics will be required, the epidural route is preferred. If contamination of an intrathecal system occurs, meningitis will result. Under normal circumstances, if this

Table 7–1. Considerations favoring implantable delivery systems

1. Likely survival greater than 2–3 months
2. Patient convenience (i.e., showering, no catheter care)
3. Good support personnel for injection schedule
4. Expense not a limiting issue
5. Recurrent percutaneous catheter dislodgement
6. Desire to use intrathecal route

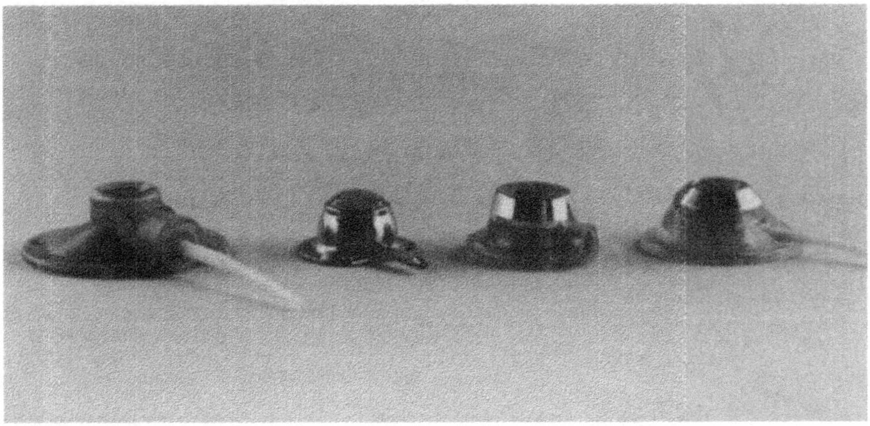

Figure 7–3. Representative sample of implantable ports marketed for chronic vascular access; however, all of them can be adapted for epidural or intrathecal drug delivery. From left to right: Infusaport, Shiley–Infusaid, Inc., Norwood, MA; Therex Implantable Port, Therex Corp., Walpole, MA; Chemport, HDC Corp., Mountain View, CA; and Mediport, Cormed, Inc., Medina, NY.
Note that systems vary according to 1) septum size, 2) profile, 3) internal and catheter dead space, 4) septum puncture tolerance, 5) weight and construction of material, i.e., titanium, polymer, stainless steel, etc., 6) mechanism for catheter attachment, and 7) design for anchoring base to tissues.

were to occur, immediate removal of the system would be required. However, since the patient's disease is generally terminal in the case of implanted systems, some clinicians have chosen to treat the infection intensely with both systemic antibiotics and intrathecal antibiotics via the implanted system. Sometimes the infection can be eradicated and the system sterilized and preserved intact. This is a difficult judgment call and is best handled in consultation with other specialists and the patient's family.

Implanted ports

To date, no vascular injection port is approved and marketed specifically for spinal drug administration. A variety of vascular access ports can be configured for spinal drug delivery. A representative though not inclusive sample of such systems is show in figure 7–3. One technical limitation of most systems used epidurally is immediately obvious. With the exception of the HDC system (Chemport), which snaps into the port, most ports either require a catheter connector or suture of the catheter onto a stem in order to attach the port to the epidural catheter (once implanted and tunnelled) to the port itself. A variety of connectors exist to link the port with the catheter. Once connected, the port is anchored at three or four points along its perimeter to the fascia, usually on the chest wall. Figure 7–4 shows a patient with a chronic

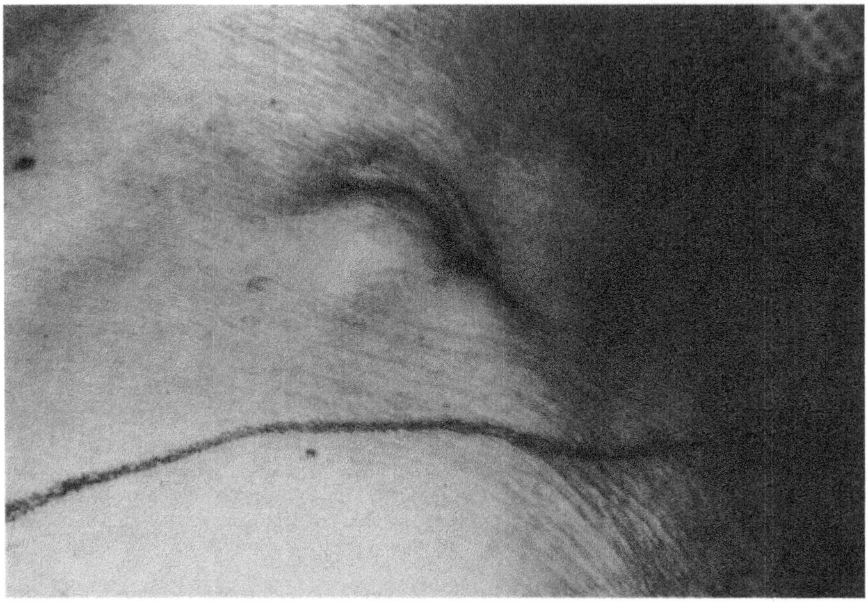

Figure 7–4. Patient with a chronic subcutaneous port attached to a thoracic epidural catheter for epidural narcotic and local anesthetic analgesia. Dark line deliniates the superior margin of the left 9th rib (lef above is posterior chest wall; anterior chest and abdomen are to the right). The subcutaneous port is located over the 7th and 8th ribs just anterior to the anterior axillary line, slightly too far posterior for optimal patient comfort with self-injection. The port had been in place for four months at the time of the photograph. No evidence of skin deterioration was encountered during six months of therapy.

thoracic epidural and attached subcutaneous port in the anterior chest position. The skin over the port is well perserved despite a TID injection regimen for most of five months.

Some comments are appropriate specifically regarding the use of subcutaneous ports, whether intrathecal or epidural. Important characteristics of the ideal port are shown in table 7–2.

An implanted port with spinal catheter has several advantages. Theoretically, the risk of infection once the system is mature should be less than with percutaneous catheters. This theory is undocumented so far. The system is more convenient in terms of wound care, showers, etc. Furthermore, the system retains the advantages of percutaneous catheters, except that continuous delivery for all but short periods is nearly impossible. Both implanted pumps and percutaneous catheters can be used with continuous flow delivery [3, 6]. The tip location of the epidural catheter is made with the same considerations as for percutaneous catheters.

The pattern of spinal narcotic delivery per epidural port is bolus intermittent

Table 7–2. Optimal characteristics of implantable ports

1. Easily palpable but not disfiguring
2. Nonreactive
3. Easy to anchor
4. Leak-resistant septum
5. Large septum area to facilitate injection
6. Small dead volume in port and catheter (less than 1/2 ml)
7. Reliable; simple to attach connection system

injection. This has the disadvantage of producing systemic redistribution of drugs [14]. However, local anesthetic use is possible if needed. In a further modification, two epidural or an epidural and an intrathecal catheter can be placed with attachment of tunnelled catheters to opposite ends of a dual port. Such a system is quite malleable. For instance, local anesthetic may be given into one dermatomal region with even a different schedule of administration for a second intrathecal or epidural agent.

Despite obvious advantages of this system under many conditions, the patient is locked into one or more daily punctures. Complications include puncture-associated discomfort, back pain upon injection, risk of infection and hemorrhage, the need for someone trained to inject the system, leakage, and failure or blockage of the system. Obstruction, kinking, and dislodgement of the catheter are all possible. The skin overlying the port may break down from infection, bleeding, puncture injury, or internal pressure erosion by the port. In practice, most of these problems are uncommon and manageable although not trivial from the standpoint of the individual requiring removal. In addition to these potential difficulties, administration personnel must be well trained and properly scheduled to accomplish ongoing deliver. Spouses and visiting nurses most commonly perform this task, although occasionally the patient can accomplish it.

Despite these limitations and adversities, the merits of this approach bear comparison with implanted infusion system, although such comparison is often difficult. Once again the major considerations are the following: 1) patterns of delivery and agents required, 2) expense of the system, and 3) support systems available. If constant spinal delivery is required to avoid bolus blood levels, then a percutaneous system with external infusion pump or an implanted infusion reservoir are the only practical alternatives. The need for local anesthetic largely precludes implanted pump use [15].[1]

Outpatient or same-day surgical placement of percutaneous or implanted system is theoretically feasible, with the understanding meticulous septic precaution is required. One must be doubly cautious about precise catheter localization (fluoroscopy with water-soluble contrast dye is recommended), since the security of close observation for infection and respiratory depression during the initial postoperative period is lost. Expense is understandably greater with the more sophisticated implantable devices. The relative cost escalates from less than $250 for the more expensive percutaneous catheters, to $350–$700 for implantable ports, to $2500–$10,000 and over for implantable pumps. Practically, if the duration of projected survival is less than four to six months, most clinicians conclude that implanted pump use is difficult to rationalize. However, patients in a remote location with minimal support systems may be well treated with an implantable pump.

Implantation

Implantation of chronic systems can be viewed as having three steps: placement of spinal catheter, creation of a pocket for reservoir or port, and tunnelling and connection of the catheter and device. Fortunately, this procedure can usually be accomplished under local or regional anesthesia using a needle technique [4]. Rarely, minilaminectomy is required [5]. Thorough skin preparation and prophylactic antibiotics are essential. Proper site location for the port/pump receptor site requires an evaluation of the skin, estimated device proximity to ostomies or wounds, and consideration of the quality and deterioration of the patient's integument. Pumps and ports should be placed in order to facilitate location by palpation but to avoid inconvenience and skin breakdown. For instance, a low anterior chest location may help a patient accomplish self-injection of a port; conversely, placement of devices too posteriorly in the flank prevents self-injection. Improper location of a pump on the abdomen may result in repetitive discomfort from belts or clothes, rubbing of the device on iliac crest (if low) or rib cage (if high). A port with a small–low-profile septum, if deeply implanted in subcutaneous tissues, will lead to frustration and failure in obese patients. In contrast, choice of a high-profile system placed in a subclavian location may succeed better. The same high-profile system may erode through the skin in an emaciated patient.

Intrathecal catheterization for chronic delivery requires modifications from standard catheter implantation techniques to prevent or limit pericatheter leakage of CSF [16, 17]. Several complications may arise. Figure 7–5 shows a patient with a small subcutaneous (CSF) hygroma or pseudomeningocoele resulting from leakage along a chronic intrathecal catheter. More serious leakage may lead to subcutaneous collections of several hundred milliliters of CSF. A chronic low-pressure headache may also result. In three cases at our clinic, an epidural blood patch reversed this phenomenon. Rarely, surgical closure of the defect may be required if only to reduce the risk of meningitis. Serious complications may arise due to low CSF pressure, including neurological deficits such as cranial nerve palsy, or subdural hematoma. These complications emphasize the need for prevention or early treatment. To this end, a simple technique can be used both to anchor the catheter from dislodgement and to reduce CSF leakage. A simple figure-eight stitch in the supraspinous ligament, placed prior to placement of the catheter, will accomplish both ends [16, 17]. The stitch is placed widely and broadly so that, when tied, the soft tissues compress the space around the catheter. The cathe-

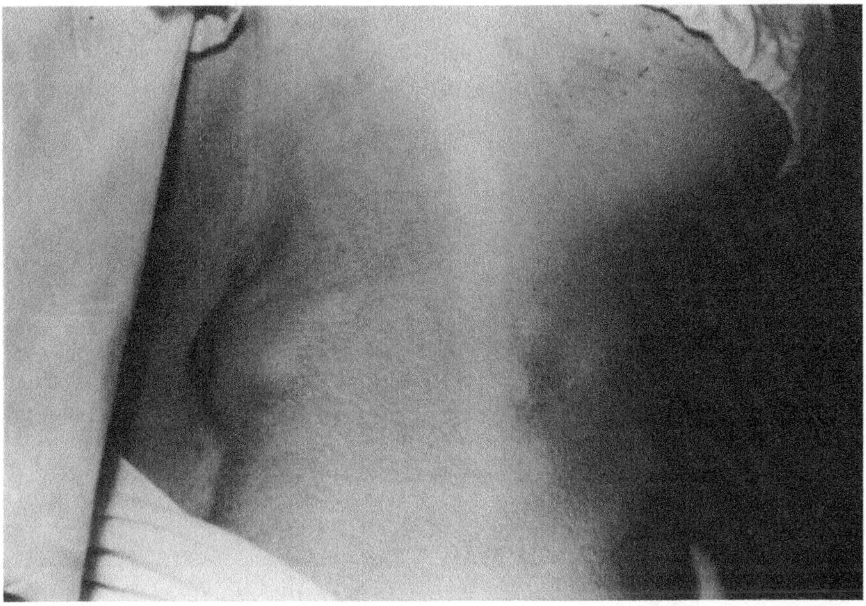

Figure 7–5. Patient receiving chronic intrathecal morphine infusion. The bulge over the lumbar spine is a CSF collection (pseudomeningocoele) from a pericatheter leak. Bedrest and a 20–ml epidural blood patch led to closure of the leak and reabsorption of the fluid.

ter is then retied to the initial knot rather than anchored and compressed with an all-encompassing tie. This simple step has eliminated our problem with CSF leaks. Presumably enough reaction eventually ensues between pericatheter tissues and silicone catheter to seal the tract.

Implantable reservoirs for spinal drug delivery

Implantable reservoirs represent the highest level of sophistication available in delivery technology, as shown in figure 7–6. This subject was reviewed in two recent monographs and has the most restricted applicability of the spinal delivery system. For this reason, only an overview of available systems will be represented along with a discussion of their advantages and disadvantages.

Implantable reservoirs can be classified into three types: patient-activated reservoirs, continuous flow systems, and programmable pumps [1, 4]. In 1981, Poletti and colleagues configured a reservoir from a blood bag and attached a compressible shunt valve in line to provide a simple patient-activated delivery system [4]. Recently Gestin completed a clinical trial in 30 patients implanted with a reservoir with buttons on its surface (Secor–Cordis Europa), allowing patient self-activated drug delivery from the system [18]. This system, shown in figure 7–6A, has a 12-ml internal reservoir, a septum

A

B

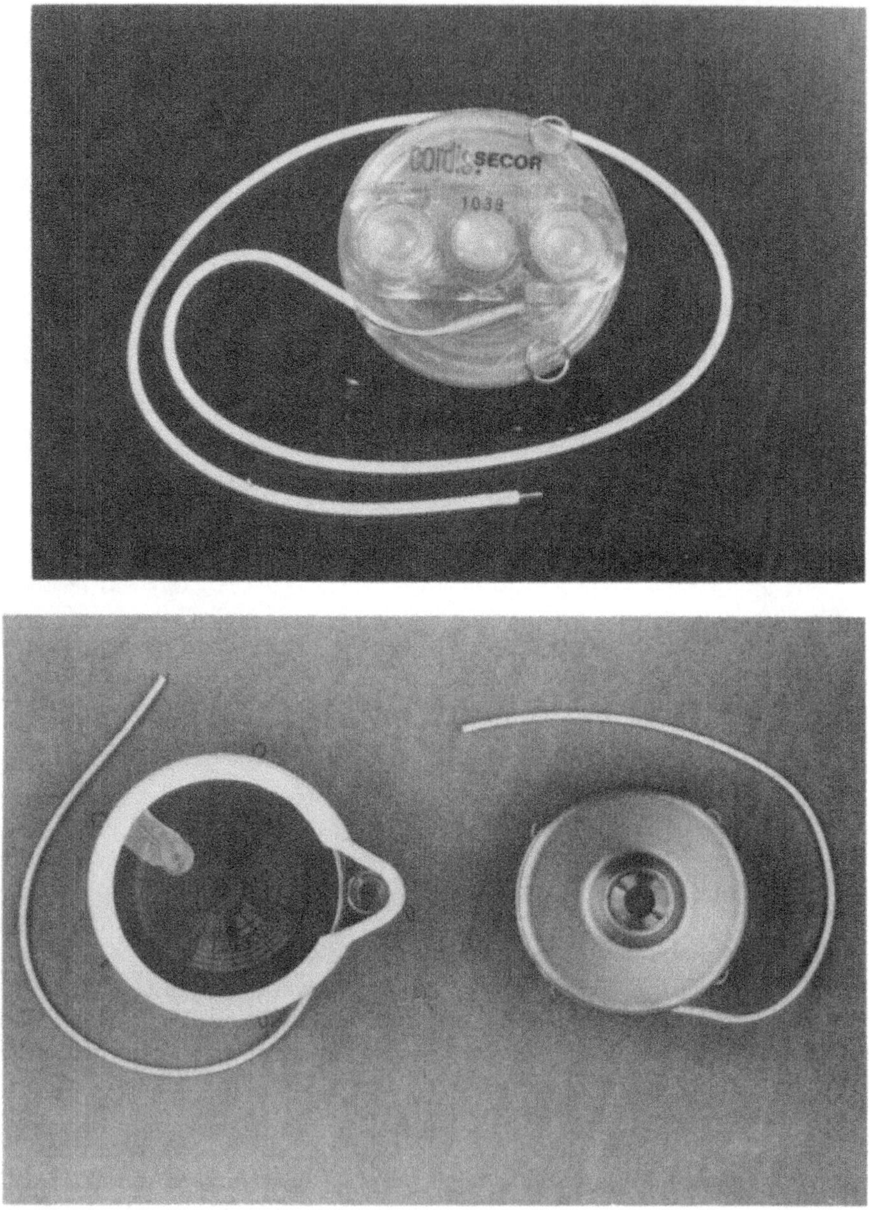

Figure 7–6. Three representative implantable reservoir drug systems.
A: The Cordis Europa Secor system, a patient-activated reservoir that delivers drug when the buttons on the front are sequentially activated correctly by the patient; delivery is by microbolus (Cordis Corp, Miami, FL).
B: Left: The Shiley–Infusaid Model 400 continuous flow pump with a single auxiliary side port. (Shiley–Infusaid, Inc., Norwood, MA.) Right: The Therex Implantable pump, a continuous flow reservoir. (Therex Corp., Walpole, MA.)

for percutaneous refill, and two buttons that must be sequentially compressed properly to eject drug from the reservoir. Obvously, the pattern of delivery is microinjection (120 boluses of 0.1 ml). The patient has responsibility for dosing unless a spouse or nurse delivers the scheduled drug. Many of the punctures associated with implanted ports are avoided, and theoretically the patient can respond quickly to increased pain without resort to systemic medication. However, there is a greater tendency perhaps for significant plasma levels of narcotic following the bolus. Further, inadvertent or intentional overdosing are possible, since the patient controls the dose schedule. In practice these problems should be rare, since cancer pain patients are usually tolerant to narcotics from prior narcotic intake. Suicide is always a risk when patients self-administer drugs and should not influence the decision to use this type of system. The projected cost may be as low as $1500 to $2000

Continuous infusion systems are another alternative. Figure 7–6B shows two systems, the first the Infusaid implantable pump, and the second the new Therex implantable pump. The Infusaid system shown here was the first implantable pump used for central nervous system drug infusion, both intrathecally and epidurally [3, 4]. Both systems in the simplest format are fixed-rate continuous-flow pumps requiring refill roughly every two to four weeks. Dose changes are accomplished by recharging the reservoirs with a different concentration of agent. Increased pain experienced by the patient often must be modulated by systemic analgesics until a reservoir concentration can be changed. The propellant for drug delivery is a freon-type fluorocarbon that generates substantial vapor pressure (about 428 mmHg at body temperature) against a metal bellows drug chamber. The drug exits through a filter system into a capillary restrictor that ultimately controls flow rate. Though temperature, barometic pressure, and viscosity theoretically effect flow rate, in practice, changes in altitude, fever, and high drug concentration have little impact on therapy. Variation in flow is about 10%–20% at the extremes encountered clinically with these factors.

Several comments about continuous flow systems are important. First, intermittent local anesthetic injection is commonly required, especially with epidural systems [16, 17]. Thus, we advocate use of pumps with an auxiliary port system, such as the Infusaid Model 400 shown. Thus this system can be either a bolus port or continuous flow pump. Second, cost of the systems (projected at about $2000 for the Therex and $4400 for the Infusaid) may decide the choice over a programmable pump system ($6000–$10000).

If continuous flow is used, should the catheter be intrathecal or epidural? Our preliminary experience indicated no difference in clinical outcome between intrathecal or epidural infusion [16]. Krames and colleagues found that some patients who could not be controlled by epidural infusion did respond to intrathecal infusion [19]. This result may be a factor of epidural fibrosis with poor drug penetration, inadequate dosage escalation, or catheter migration; or intrathecal delivery may indeed be better. This question remains unanswered.

The choice of spinal analgesic, over and above local anesthetics, may dictate the delivery system chosen. Morphine has been the primary agent for continuous infusion. Stability and compatibility data on other drugs, as well as chronic neurotoxicity data, do not exist for most implanted systems [7]. Some clinical experience exists with hydromorphone, but chronic data are lacking with the newer anilino-4-piperidine narcotics, buprenorphine, and other synthetic agents [20]. The delta opioid receptor-specific peptide, DADLE, and the alpha$_2$, adrenergic agonist, clonidine, have both undergone preliminary trials, but neither is approved by the FDA [20–22]. Thus approved pharmacology is limited for use with these systems. Individualized therapy in the event of analgesic failure is facilitated with percutaneous and port systems, since no risk of pump failure exists. In contrast, new drugs to be tried in implantable systems may yield electrolytic effects with internal components of the pump, precipitate and obstruct the system, degrade the filter, be unstable, or undergo breakdown to an altogether different and perhaps toxic drug or metabolite. Unfortunately, expanding pharmacology in this area is a difficult, expensive, and time-consuming exercise [7].

The third implantable alternative is a programmable pump such as the Medtronic pump. Shiley Infusaid, Minimed, and Siemens have all developed similar systems with many overlapping features. Common to all is a high projected price, generally in excess of $6000. Two components are needed, the pump itself and a radiofrequency programmer, similar to the units required to reprogram implanted cardiac pacemakers. Systems such as the Medtronic pump can be programmed to deliver variable flow rates, pulses, continuous flow, and other patterns of flow. In preliminary studies, Penn et al. could not demonstrate an advantage of such a system in this application [23]. Theoretically, the patient could program a change if pain increased or disappeared and telephone monitoring could be used both to assess the status of the system and to recommend programming changes to the patient. Another considerable factor, over and above the complexity and expense of the systems, is the need to replace the pump batteries, in some cases in less than three years. In terms of spinal narcotic delivery, this fact is of pragmatic significance only in a case of therapy to control spasticity in spinal-cord-injured patients [24].

The last point to be made is the issue of who should implant and manage such systems. On the face of it, anesthesiologists or neurosurgeons could place such systems, functioning strictly in a technical capacity. However, proper decisions about the choice of an appropriate system can only be made by a clinician familiar with the pharmacology of cancer pain and related analgesic techniques. Also required is a thorough understanding of spinal neuropharmacology, implantable systems, and their complications, and perhaps equally importantly, a network to support the patient once the system is in place. The latter is of necessity a demanding, time-consuming exercise. Our experience has *convinced* us that a collaborative system is the best course if possible and that a qualified neurosurgeon is an invaluable member of the team. Up to implanting reservoirs, an anesthesiologist can perform all the intellectual and technical facets of chronic spinal analgesic therapy. Some of the complications and indeed the spinal implantation of catheters in certain anatomical situations will require the surgical skills of a neurosurgeon, i.e., repair of CSF leaks, minilaminectomy for spinal catheter placement, and treatment of serious epidural and pump pocket infections. Furthermore, some patients will fail spinal analgesic therapy and require cordotomies or other palliative procedures to relieve pain.

CONCLUSIONS

The clinician has available a variety of implements to deliver spinal analgesics. These tools should be viewed in context. They are, in fact, a small but important part of applied spinal neuropharmacology. Such technology will no doubt become increasingly important as applied neuropharmacology expands into nonmalignant pain, spasticity, and other applications [7].

ACKNOWLEDGMENTS

This work and Dr. Coombs' time in editing this volume have been supported in part by PHS grant CA-33865 of the NCI, as well as by funds from the Robert Osgood Jr. Memorial Fund and the Kingsburg Fund.

NOTES

1. Kroin et al. [15] report chronic intrathecal bupivacaine infusion in dogs, suggesting that this may be feasible for implanted pumps; notably, a prior clinical trial with chronic *epidural* bupivacaine infusion at our institution was largely unsuccessful using implanted infusion reservoirs. (Coombs DW, et al. 1982. Intraspinal narcotic-tolerance. Int J Artific Organs 5:379–382).

REFERENCES

1. Coombs DW. 1986. Management of chronic pain by epidural and intrathecal opioids: Newer drugs and delivery systems. In Sjöstrand UH, Rawal N (eds): Regional Opioids in Anesthesiology and Pain Management. Int Anesthesiol Clin 24:59–74.
2. Coombs DW. 1985. New approaches to chronic pain therapy. Semin Anesthesia 4:287–299.
3. Coombs DW, Saunders RL, Gaylor M, et al. 1982. Epidural narcotic infusion reservoir: Implantation technique and efficacy. Anesthesiology 56:469–473.
4. Poletti CE, Cohen AM, Todd DP, Ojeman RE, et al. 1981. Cancer pain relieved by long term epidural morphine with permanent indwelling systems for self administration. J Neurosurg 55:581–584.
5. Onofrio BM, Yaksh TL, Arnold PE. 1981. Continuous low-dose intrathecal morphine administration in the treatment of chronic pain of malignant origin. Mayo Clinic Proc 56:516–520.
6. Mather LE, Raj PP. 1986. Spinal opiates. In Raj PP (ed): Practical Management of Pain. Chicago: Year Book Medical Publishers, Inc., pp. 709–727.
7. Coombs DW, Fratkin JD. 1987. Neurotoxicity of spinal agents. Anesthesiology 66:724–725.
8. Coombs DW, Fratkin JD, Meier F, et al. 1985. Neuropathologic lesions and CSF morphine concentrations during chronic continuous intraspinal morphine infusion: A clinical and post mortem study. Pain 22:337–351.
9. Coombs DW. 1988. Intraspinal analgesic Infusion by Implanted Pump. In Penn, RD (ed): Neurological Applications of Implanted Drug Pumps. Ann Ny Acad Sci 531:108–122.
10. Roda BA, Cohen FL, Bean WJ, Martyak SN., 1985. Fibrous mass complicating epidural morphine infusion. Neurosurgery 16:68–70.

11. Zenz M. 1984. Epidural opiates for the treatment of cancer pain. In Zimmerman M, Drugs P, Wagner G (eds): Recent Results in Cancer Research Vol. 89. Heidelberg: Springer Verlag, pp. 107–115.
12. Eriksen J, Andersen HB. 1984. Pain treatment on long term basis using extradural opiates. Pain (Suppl 2) 19:S335.
13. DuPenn SL, Peterson DE, Bogosian AC, Ramsey DH, Larsonc, Omoto M. 1987. A new permanent exteriorized epidural cutheter for narcotic self-administration of control cancer pain. Cancer 59:986–993.
14. Cousins MJ, Mather LE. 1984. Intrathecal and epidural administration of opiates. Anesthesiology 61:276–310.
15. Kroin JS, Mc Carthy RJ, Penn RD, Kerns JM, Ivankovich AD. 1987. The effect of chronic subarachnoid bupivacaine in fusion in dogs, anesthesiology 66:737–742.
16. Coombs DW, Maurer LH, Saunders RL, Jensen LE. 1984. Outcomes and complications of continuous intraspinal narcotic analgesia for cancer pain control. J Clin Oncol 2:1414–1420.
17. Coombs DW. 1985. Continuous Spinal Morphine Analgesia for Relief of Cancer Pain. Cambridge, MA: Shea Bros., pp. 1–29.
18. Gestin Y. 1987. A totally implantable multi-dose pump allowing cancer patients intrathecal access for the self administration of morphine at home. A follow up of 30 cases. Der Anaesthetist 36:391.
19. Krames ES, Gershow J, Glassberg A, Kenefick T, Lyons A, et al. 1985. Continuous infusion of spinally administered narcotics for the relief of pain due to malignant disorders. Cancer 56:692–702.
20. Coombs DW, Saunders RL, Fratkin JD, et al. 1986. Continuous intrathecal hydromorphine and clonidine for intractable cancer pain. J Neurosurg 64:890–894.
21. Onofrio BM, Yaksh TL. 1983. Intrathecal delta-receptor ligand produces analgesia in man. Lancet i:1386.
22. Coombs DW, Saunders RL, LaChance D, Savage S, et al. 1985. Intrathecal morphine tolerance: Use of intrathecal clonidine, DADL, and intraventricular morphine. Anesthesiology 62:358–363.
23. Penn RD, Paice JA, Gottschalk W, Ivankovich A. 1984. Cancer pain relief using chronic morphine infusion. J Neurosurg 61:302–306.
24. Erickson DL, Blacklock JB, Michaelson M, et al. 1985. Control of spasticity by implantable continuous flow morphine pump. Neurosurgery 16:215–217.

8. SPINAL OPIOID ANALGESIA: PRESENT STATUS AND FUTURE DEVELOPMENTS

PERRY G. FINE AND THEODORE H. STANLEY

Recognition of opiate binding sites (receptors) in the dorsal horn of the spinal cord rapidly led to the demonstration of spinal opioid-mediated analgesia [1–3] and new techniques for delivering pain relief [4–6]. The capability of blocking nociception at discrete spinal cord receptor sites without motor, sensory, or sympathetic blockade is a quantum step forward in pain management. Furthermore, the potential exists for even more precise localization of active receptor sites in the spinal cord, which could dramatically change conventional approaches of administering many times the dose of a drug to effect "equivalent" analgesia. Such changes could eliminate or drastically reduce systemic and other undesirable side effects of oral, parenteral, or spinal analgesia (anesthesia). Thus, spinal opioid analgesia (SOA) may serve as a model for a new principle of anesthetic drug administration that we shall call *drug focusing*.

In spite of all the superlatives, SOA is not yet without significant limitations. In acute care settings, i.e., postoperative and trauma pain relief, SOA can cause delayed and sometimes profound respiratory depression. Less severe but more frequent problems include pruritus, urinary retention, and nausea. In patients with chronic pain (from malignancy), development of tolerance and the unavailability of safe, reliable, inexpensive delivery systems are still significant obstacles. In addition, knowledge of the pharmacodynamics, pharmacokinetics, and the importance of receptor kinetics of drugs delivered by the spinal route is incomplete, as are the long-term effects of such agents on neural tissue. As a result the search for the "ideal drug" and method of delivery for spinal analgesia continues.

This chapter will highlight present and future research on the above issues. Epidural versus subarachnoid routes of administration will be viewed independently, since the factors of dose, volume, concentration, distribution, uptake, and disposition are often different. Developments in analgesia mediated by nonopioids and their interactions with the spinal opioid system will also be addressed. We will conclude with a discussion of emerging concepts of *drug focusing* and *energetic perturbation* as applied to spinal analgesia and, more generally, to anesthesiology as a whole.

PRESENT RESEARCH

Selective spinal analgesia by epidural administration of morphine was first reported [7, 8] shortly after Wang et al. [3] demonstrated the efficacy of intrathecal morphine for pain relief in patients with cancer. Numerous confirmatory reports followed, and the entire subject was summarized by Cousins in 1984 [6]. Since that time other investigators have attempted to understand the pharmacodynamics and pharmacokinetics of the numerous volumes, concentrations, and differing types of opioids being delivered to the spinal axis at multiple sites. Respiratory depression continues to be the most severe and feared complication of techniques that administer opioids to the epidural or intrathecal spaces. Factors contributing to this problem, including rostral spread of the drug to supraspinal respiratory centers via cerebrospinal fluid (CSF) redistribution or vascular uptake and systemic absorption, are being explored, and considerable advances in understanding have been made.

The cumulative data lead us to conclude that drugs for spinal analgesia should readily cross the dura (when administered in the epidural space); should be lipophilic and thus rapidly enter the spinal cord; should possess a high affinity for receptors mediating opioid analgesia (mu, kappa, delta); should be associated with minimal or no risk or systemic effects; should cause minimal tolerance or cross-tolerance; should have no effect on bladder or bowel function; and should result in no tissue toxicity. Although most clinicians have used morphine for SOA, it is clearly not the ideal drug for these techniques. The following sections will highlight directions and results of the most recent investigations of SOA.

The epidural route

Absorption and distribution

It is now well established that morphine administered in the epidural space is absorbed by epidural blood vessels at sufficient rates to produce plasma concentrations equal to those occurring when the same dose is given intramuscularly [9, 10]. Studies of other opioids reveal that the more lipophilic the drug, the more rapidly and completely systemic absorption occurs. Thus, similar systemic effects as occur following more traditional parenteral approaches should be anticipated, and appropriate observation/monitoring ensured before instituting epidural opioid techniques.

The hypothesis that *delayed* respiratory depression after epidural administration of an opioid is due to cephalad migration (intrathecal ascent) is now well established [11]. It is also clear that this problem is significantly more likely after administration of a hydrophilic opioid (e.g., morphine) than a more lipid-soluble compound (e.g., fentanyl). This observation indicates that cephalad migration is the probable explanation of why morphine given at a lumbar epidural level will result in analgesia at higher (thoracic or even cervical) levels [12–14].

Effects of volume

The volume of a hydrophilic agent in the epidural space is not an important influence on the height (spread) of analgesia or duration of action. The most frequently offered explanation for this observation is that hydrophilic drugs remain in the CSF for a prolonged period after dural penetration, allowing for redistribution throughout the subarachnoid space, and thus minimizing volume effects. In contrast, lipophilic agents such as fentanyl and methadone penetrate the dura with ease and bind rapidly to neural tissue. Since their residence within the CSF is relatively brief, increasing the volume of an injectate of these substances leads to higher segmental levels of spinal analgesia [15]. Additional studies with other agents more and less lipid-soluble than morphine and fentanyl would be helpful in confirming these early observations and theories regarding the importance of volume on the spread of analgesia. Changes in epidural pressure also seems to cause minimal changes in the spread of analgesia after epidural opioid administration [16]. Although there is a direct correlation between volume infused and epidural-space pressure, the maximum pressure attained with up to 35 ml/hr of fentanyl in a saline solution is neither physiologically nor clinically remarkable [16]. Thus it appears that with the usual volumes of epidural solutions employed, epidural space-pressure change is not a variable of any clinical consequence.

Dose–response relationships

DURATION. A number of recent postoperative studies have established a strong positive dose–response relationship for duration and magnitude of epidural opioid analgesia. A strong correlation between increasing dose and side effects (nausea, vomiting, pruritus, urinary retention, and respiratory depression) is also described with epidural opioids. These relationships do not seem to be appreciably influenced by the operative site, since results have been similar in controlled studies involving orthopedic lower-extremity procedures [17], peripheral vascular operations [18], and thoracotomy [12]. Although individual variation is always important, most studies suggest that 3–5 mg of morphine will provide adequate analgesia lasting for approximately 12 hours in adults with pain from somatosomes below the cervical level.

Vasoconstrictors, which are commonly used to prolong the duration of subarachnoid local anesthetics but are less effective in local anesthetic epidural blocks, are also ineffective in prolonging analgesia from epidural opioids. Parker et al. found that adding epinephrine to epidurally administered fentanyl, sufentanil, or hydromorphone did not alter the duration of analgesia [19].

VENTILATORY EFFECTS. Ventilatory effects of epidural morphine have been recently studied in patients after cholecystectomy operations and health volunteers. Rawal and Wattwil [20] evaluated the effects of 2-, 4-, and 10-mg doses of epidural morphine on the ventilatory function of both groups of subjects over 22-hour periods. End-tital CO_2 ($ETCO_2$) and minute ventilation responses to increases in inspired CO_2 were measured following epidural administration of morphine. Patients that had received a general anesthetic for cholecystectomy prior to epidural morphine had a dose-related increase in $ETCO_2$ and a diminished response to increases in inspired CO_2 compared with volunteers receiving epidural morphine alone. These findings suggest that spinal opioids potentiate residual central nervous system depression following general anesthesia. Respiratory rates of postsurgical subjects did not correlate with measured $ETCO_2$ levels; in spite of normal or elevated respiratory rates, $ETCO_2$ remained elevated. These results indicate that respiratory rate is not a reliable means of monitoring ventilatory adequacy in postoperative patients. Furthermore, it was demonstrated that 4 mg of epidural morphine did not cause *clinically signficant* respiratory depression in adults with otherwise normal ventilatory function.

Other investigators have demonstrated similar changes in $PaCO_2$ for up to three hours after intramuscular or epidural administration of 200 mcg of fentanyl following thoracic or upper abdominal procedures [21]. However, forced vital capacity (FVC) was improved by 22% along with a 25% decrease in respiratory rate the first hour after epidural fentanyl as compared with intramuscular fentanyl. These data clearly demonstrate improved ventilatory efficiency with epidural fentanyl compared with an equivalent dose of intramuscular fentanyl.

METABOLISM. There are few published date on the effects of opioids on spinal cord metabolism [22]. However, such effects may be of clinical importance because down-regulation of metabolic activity may be associated with reduced permanent neurologic damage after spinal cord injury or surgery. Lin and coworkers have recently demonstrated that epidural fentanyl decreases spinal cord metabolic rate (measured by glucose metabolism) in a rat model [23]. The mechanism(s) involved have not yet been elucidated.

Delivery systems

A number of investigators have explored the possibility of prolonged epidural opioid analgesia by employing a catheter in the epidural space for repeated injection [24]. In addition, a variation of the patient-controlled analgesia

(PCA) technique has been described by Chrubasik and Wiemers [25]. Using a small, externally worn infusion device, these authors have shown that patients can self-regulate their epidural dose of morphine after abdominal surgery to optimize analgesia. These patients' total daily narcotic intake continually decreased over the postoperative period without ever compromising analgesia. The authors reported no complications.

Raj et al. showed that continuous epidural opioid analgesia reduced hospital stay after knee surgery [26]. Patients reported better analgesia and as a result reduced their hospital stay an average of four days compared to patients provided conventional parenteral narcotics. Savings in terms of direct inpatient costs and nosocomial risks were not calculated, but must have been substantial. Cost–benefit research of this nature will likely continue to be of interest and considerable value.

The intrathecal route

Distribution

A number of animal models have now been devised that serve as useful predictors of human CSF dynamics and can be employed to evaluate opioid distribution patterns after injection into the subarachnoid space. Gustafsson et al. have used whole-body autoradiography to follow the distribution of radioisotope-labeled opioids injected into the intrathecal space of rats [27]. They found that morphine remained within the sinal cord in greater concentration at 14 and 44 minutes after injection compared with meperidine, a more lipophilic opioid. These data support the thesis that redistribution of intrathecal opioid away from the spinal axis is correlated to lipid solubility. This model would also be useful to study distribution effects from changes in volume, concentration, and molecular weight of different opioids injected into the CSF.

Payne and Inturrisi have used a sheep preparation to determine lumbar to cisternal movement of drugs [28]. They have shown that (hydrophilic) morphine moves in a cephalad direction more rapidly (between 90 and 190 minutes) than (lipophilic) methadone (greater than 240 minutes). Others [29] have shown that approximately 67% of methadone but only 3.8% of morphine is absorbed by the spinal cord minutes after intrathecal injection. Obviously much of the remaining morphine is available for subsequent extraspinal redistribution, or spinal or supraspinal uptake. The information obtained from these studies compares well with clinical observations made using intrathecal morphine and methadone and appears useful in predicting the clinical activity of other potentially useful drugs for spinal analgesia.

Dose–Response

Clinicians evaluating intrathecal opioids have employed a considerable range of doses. A study by Glass et al. [30] lends some insight into the issue of the *appropriate dose* of morphine (presently the only commercially available opioid specifically designated for spinal use in the U.S.A.). They report that four-fold dose differences of intrathecal morphine (0.1–0.4 mg) result in similar degrees (magnitude and duration) of postoperative analgesia, respiratory changes ($PaCO_2$, FEV_1, peak flow, FVC), and side effects. With additional studies (with morphine and other drugs delivered intrathecally) it may be possibly to generate predictable dose–response curves, allowing optimization of therapeutic effect and minimization of side effects.

Some investigators have suggested that intravenous opioid antagonists can minimize or reverse side effects without affecting SOA. Daily et al. compared naloxone and saline (administered as an infusion) in laboring women after a 1-mg dose of intrathecal morphine [31]. They found that naloxone (0.4 mg as an intravenous bolus followed by a 0.4–0.6 mg/hr infusion) alleviated pruritus but had no effect on dizziness, somnolence, and urinary retention. Their results demonstrate that intravenous naloxone is a safe and effective antagonist for pruritus. Unfortunately they could not explain why the other side effects were not affected. Since there was no control group (placebo intrathecal injection or non-SOA group), conclusions regarding the cause of nonreversible side effects could not be further evaluated. Dose–response relationships of spinal opioid antagonism by naloxone and other narcotic reversal agents remain unclear.

Neurotoxicity

There is a paucity of long-term studies analyzing the histopathologic consequences of applying opioids to the tissues of the neuroaxis. Nonetheless, few if any problems have been reported. In their recent review article, Cousins and Mather [6] found no supporting evidence of spinal cord pathology in animals or man after spinal administration of morphine.

Most recently, Coombs et al. report findings from postmortem studies of seven patients with terminal cancer after chronic administration of intrathecal morphine [32]. Posterior column degeneration was found in two of the patients, though specific clinical symptoms or signs were not noted before death. The etiology of these changes (whether primarily related to disease, treament modalities, or analgesia administration) remains obscure even after thorough retrospective review by the authors. It seems unlikely that the lesions were caused by the delivery system or spinal morphine; however, the use of intrathecal opioids must continue to be carefully evaluated.

Specific agents

There is as yet no single agent that fulfills all critieria for the "ideal" spinal analgesic. Numerous compounds, some old and some quite newly developed, have been recently tested. This section will attempt to elucidate some of the unique characteristics and properties of the compounds thus far evaluated.

Selective opioid agonists

DIACETYLMORPHINE. Because of its lipid solubility and metabolic fate, diacetylmorphine (heroin) has been evaluated for epidural and intrathecal application in a number of studies. Heroin is 17 times more soluble in fat than water and is thus readily absorbed into neural tissues [33]. Once in neural tissue, heroin undergoes deacetylation to its principal metabolite, morphine, which is hydrophilic. Thus, when placed in the epidural or intrathecal space, very little of the parent compound remains free to redistribute in the CSF; but once in the spinal cord, clearance is relatively slow [34, 35]. Spinal use of diacetylmorphine should afford long-lasting analgesia (like morphine) with low risk of latent supraspinal effects, particularly respiratory depression. The debate (mostly emotional and political) concerning legalization of heroin in North America notwithstanding [36], the cumulative data regarding its utility for SOA seem to represent a scientific basis for the theory that heroin may have a clinically advantageous role.

METHADONE. Methadone has a relatively long half-life when given orally or parenterally and may be useful in clinical settings where prolonged analgesia is a benefit [37]. In contrast, it has limited utility for SOA because its lipid solubility leads to rapid clearance and a short duration of action after a single dose. However, a recent study by Evron et al. [38] using epidural methadone indicates that equianalgesic epidural doses of methadone caused less urinary disturbance than morphine after Caesarean section. There is, as yet, no satisfactory explanation for this difference despite the apparent similar activity of these agents at the same receptor binding sites. This study demonstrates the heterogeneity of clinical effects that members of the same opioid class of drugs manifest. It appears that these effects are not predictable from known physiochemical or pharmacokinetic properties of the drugs.

ALFENTANIL. Yaksh et al. have investigated the fentanyl congener alfentanil in a continuous subarachnoid infusion [39]. Its intrathecal kinetic profile is similar to that of fentanyl; however, alfentanil's lower volume of distribution should make systemic accumulation, which is an occasional problem with multiple doses of fentanyl, less likely with alfentanil. A lower volume of distribution allows for a steady-state level of drug delivery and activity at spinal sites without systemic effects or concern for the consequences of supraspinal redistribution. These properties, if valid after epidural or intrathecal use of alfentanil, might obviate some of the monitoring problems and hesitancy that now occurs with SOA in nonintensive care settings after operation.

ENDOGENOUS OPIOIDS. Isolation, purification, and even synthesis of some naturally occurring (endogenous) opioids have led to investigations of their use for SOA. The polypeptides beta-endorphin and dynorphin have been evaluated and appear to render potent analgesia in extremely low doses (30 μg) without appreciable ill effects following intrathecal administration [40]. Unfortunately these trials have been limited and short-term. Far more experience and information is necessary before meaningful analysis and comparisons are possible.

PARTIAL AGONISTS. The term *partial agonist* describes opioid drugs that have agonist (analgesic) activity at a specific receptor but whose effect is maximized at a given dose (above which there is no further effect). This subclass of drug may also antagonize, by competitive inhibition, other agonists acting at similar receptor (binding) sites.

Buprenorphine is a new partial agonist compound with high affinity for μ-receptor sites and has been evaluated and compared with morphine. Recent work led by Murphy [41] and Lanz [42] indicates that buprenorphine produces profound spinal analgesia and fewer side effecs than morphine. These authors found no evidence of respiratory depression. Buprenorphine is five times more lipid-soluble than morphine and has 50 times more affinity for μ-receptors than morphine [43]. These characteristics may explain why relatively small doses (60–300 ug) of buprenorphine have long-lasting effects and minimal propensity toward rostral redistribution. Studies comparing the magnitude and duration of analgesia after epidural and intravenous administration of buprenorphine with co-related blood levels of the drug are in progress [41].

U-50, 488H. The thesis that analgesia can be mediated at the spinal level by K-receptors without supraspinal respiratory center μ-receptor effects has been elaborated in a study in rats by Castillo et al. [44]. In this model, rats were given the experimental selective K-receptor agonist U-50, 488H via lumbar epidural or intracerebral ventricular catheters. Analgesia to tail clamping was evaluated after lumbar epidural dosing, and respiratory function (respiratory rate and $PaCO_2$) was measured after ventricular administration. Analgesia occurred without any ventilatory changes. The results suggest that analgesia and respiratory depression may be mediated independently and via different receptors. Combination of these data with those of investigators demonstrating increasingly selective opioid receptor agonists [45] should lead to safer clinical utilization of this valuable analgesic technique.

AGONIST–ANTAGONISTS. It is logical that a drug that might block opioid-mediated respiratory depression but would specifically promote analgesia at the spinal level would be useful and would enhance the safety of SOA. Because of μ-receptor antagonism and K- and σ-receptor agonist activity, the term *agonist–antagonist* or *mixed agonist* has been applied to drugs such as pentazocine and butorphanol. Supraspinal effects of these drugs on the K-receptor include analgesia and sedation. Stimulation of the σ-receptor causes dysphoria and other psychomimetic effects. The properties of these receptors in the spinal cord are less clear. However, Kalia and coworkers suggest that a 0.3-mg epidural dose of pentazocine provided reliable analgesia following gynecological surgery without urinary retention, pruritus, or respiratory problems [46]. Carefully controlled studies evaluating respiratory function and supraspinal redistribution, including comparisons to morphine, have been done and are necessary. It is also noteworthy that spinal administration of this class of drug has the potential for provoking an acute abstinence syndrome in narcotic-tolerant patients [47].

Opioidlike and nonopioid agents

KETAMINE. Though supraspinal analgesia from ketamine is most likely not mediated via opioid receptors [48], the discovery that ketamine binds to (nonspecified) opioid receptors [49] has led to investigations of this phencyclidine as a potential mediator of spinal analgesia. Trials thus far have been limited, but Bion noted that doses (up to 50 mg) of intrathecal ketamine in patients with recent trauma resulted in surgical analgesia [50]. Although a sensory level of analgesia was obtained and the density of the block improved with the addition of epinephrine, the effect of a single dose was short-lived (approximately 45 minutes). Bion attributed the short duration of analgesia to the purportedly high lipid solubility of ketamine. High lipid solubility may also lead to supraspinal depression due to vascular absorption and systemic redistribution. Islas et al. used epidural ketamine to control postoperative pain [51]. Though this study lacked controls and randomization, the data indicate that low doses (4 mg) of epidural ketamine provide potent analgesia with little if any side effects.

ADRENERGIC AGENTS. Recent studies in animals and man have demonstrated potentiation of opioid activity by adrenergic agonists at the spinal level. Evidence for such an interaction was provided in animal studies in which clonidine, an adrenergic (alpha-2) agonist, was shown to prevent opioid withdrawal activity when administered at spinal and supraspinal sites [52, 53].

Taiwo et al. demonstrated that serotonin and norepinephrine potentiate morphine's antinociceptive activity on the spinal cords of rats [54]. It had been hoped that synergistic antinociceptive activity of subthreshold doses of these (and other) agents could minimize adverse effects and delay the development of tolerance to opioids during long-term analgesic administration. Unfortunately, recent reports of cross-tolerance with different classes of drugs may temper the initial enthusiasm of proponents of these approaches.

That there may be interactions between opioid and adrenergic receptors resulting in cross-tolerance has been shown in a rat model by Milne et al. [55]. After demonstrating equivalent analgesia with intrathecal morphine and norepinephrine, the authors allowed tolerance to each of the agents to develop by long-term exposure to the respective drug through an indwelling intrathecal catheter. Following this, they administered the other compound and found significantly less analgesic activity than when it was first administered, i.e., cross-tolerance. Similar results were observed in man by Coombs et al. after extremely high doses of intrathecal and intraventricular morphine were administered to a patient with end-stage cancer [56]. They found that intraventricular doses of synthetic enkephalin peptide DADLE (A δ-receptor agonist) was ineffective in providing analgesia, as were increasingly high doses of intrathecal clonidine after tolerance to morphine occurred. These findings suggest that there might be little clinical utility of alternating μ-, δ-, and adrenergic spinal receptor agonists after opioid tolerance develops.

A number of representatives from various nonopioid and noncatecholamine drug classes, including several naturally occurring compounds, have been evaluated for analgesic activity at the spinal cord level. Immunocytochemical techniques have provided evidence of binding sites of many such agents within the dorsal horns of the spinal cord. Substances with such putative spinal antinociceptive activity or modulating influence include prostaglandins, vasoactive intestinal polypeptide, cholecystokinin, somatostatin, thyrotropin releasing hormone, avian pancreatic polypeptide, angiotensin II, some benzodiazepines, and the gamma-amino-butyric-acid (GABA) receptor agonist baclofen [7, 57–59].

One of the most interesting of these substances has been the polypeptide somatostatin (a hypothalamic factor that regulates pituitary release of growth hormone) [7]. Intrathecal, intraventricular, and epidural administration of somatostatin results in analgesia without side effects in rats and dogs [60]. The compound has also been evaluated for its analgesic effects in man after operation and in terminally ill patients. Somatostatin is 1.6 times as potent as epidural morphine [61] and 8 times as potent as intrathecal morphine [62]. No adverse or toxic effects have been noted in man, and this agent's analgesic activity seems to be mediated by nonopioid receptor mechanisms, for the analgesic effects are not reversible with naloxone [63]. Yaksh, has been unable to demonstrate significant analgesia in chronically spinally cannulated rats; futhermore, the compound was seriously neurotoxic in the preparation. Somatostatin is now commercially available, as is a synthetic polypeptide analogue, SMS 201–995 (Sandoz, Basel, Switzerland) [64], a parenterally long-acting agent that has been successfully used in the long-term treatment of acromegaly (suppressing growth hormone) [65]. It is difficult to speculate on the potential of spinally mediated analgesia with somatostatin or its congeners. However, refinements in delivery techniques and development of selective compounds, which can be applied or directed to specific target sites (receptors, organs, membranes) to produce circumscribed activity with minimal or no undesirable effects, exemplifies the principal advantage of drug specificity and refined drug delivery that we generically label drug focusing.

FUTURE DIRECTIONS

Drug focusing

Synthesis and refinement of opioid and nonopioid compounds have resulted in more potent congeners that are more selective in function [66]. This has been a first step in the enhancement of therapeutic activity and the simultaneous reduction of toxic effects, which has yielded drugs with greater specificity and a higher therapeutic index (LD_{50}/ED_{50}). The concept of drug focusing addresses the goal of limiting drug action to specific receptor sites within certain organs or specific tissues, and applies not only to the subject at hand (spinal analgesia) but to anesthesiology and perhaps many areas of medicine at large.

The development of liposomes, microscopic lipid bags or envelopes that can encase drugs, now provides a mechanism by which many compounds could be carried in an inactive form after injection into the blood stream [67]. Advantageous properties of liposomes for this purpose include their biodegradability and similarity to natural membranes. They can also be modified to suit a variety of compounds and situations [67–70]. The challenge now is to utilize developments in wave technology, computer-directed techniques, and photomedicine to direct and disintegrate these otherwise inert parcels. It is possible to selectively break these lipid bags by focusing microwave, ultrasonic, or other waves on them so that the temperature of the membrane of the bag is only slightly increased (perhaps 1.5–2.0 C), a temperature that will rupture the bag (B. Mills personal communication). Only the bags within the focal spectrum of the wave being utilized will break, and thus the contained drug(s) will only be released in the desired local area. It would also seem possible that laser energy could be used to selectively destroy inert liposomes carrying an active agent or cleave a bound compound so that an inactive form of an agent would become active. To the best of our knowledge this has not yet been accomplished.

Can the revolutionary developments in imaging technology be utilized to focus drugs or lipid bags containing pharmacologically active compounds at discrete sites in the central nervous system? The experts (D. Ailion personal communication) say that identification of receptors or chemical components of the receptors is plausible with a technique called high-resolution focusing. However, as of this writing, direct steering of the drug to the identified receptor is difficult. The reason appears to be related to the fact that current computer-directed imaging technologies do not steer but rather orient molecules (nuclei). Having identified both the location where the drug is to act and a means to activate the drug leaves the final problem, namely focusing the drug on the receptor. One wonders if this might not be solved by attempting to design the drug (or carrier) to be attracted to the receptor via an antigen–antibody mechanism, applying principles similar to those evolving with monoclonal antibodies [71]. Another possibility would be systemic injection of an inactive drug that is then activated by an energy source (e.g., laser) focused on the receptor site.

Drug activity without the drug

Concepts related to affecting and particularly to depressing CNS activity without use of pharmacologic compounds are not new [72]. In fact, it is possible to trace to the turn of this century the use of electrical currents for the precise purpose of producing anesthesia. Some authors have even traced these ideas back to Biblical times [72, 73]. More frequently, acupuncture and methods of producing analgesia via transcutaneous electrical stimulation have become popular and are, at least in some anesthesiologists' experience, effective in patients [74–77]. The recognition of transmitter–receptor interactions as a cause of many natural cerebral activities, the evolution of specific CNS-acting drugs that depress the spinal cord and/or brain via interference or effects on neutrotransmitters, receptors, or both, and the realization that drug and neurotransmitter action at receptor sites can be electrically provoked raises the possibility of producing drug action on the CNS (perhaps profound drug action) without need for the drug. Indeed, the ability to identify the receptor in vivo (perhaps noninvasively, utilizing computer-controlled imaging technology) suggests that it should be possible to directly affect (depress, activate, interfere with) receptor activity via focused energy sources (on the receptor). The trick now is to identify the precise (best) energy source and set of characteristics and to focus that source precisely on that part of the cell(s) membrane, so that nerve conduction may be reversibly interrupted. The power of current imaging technology as well as the availability and developing knowledge base of energy and wave sources is critical to future drug focusing. However, it is already quite clear that externally applied electrical fields can induce and/or alter polarization in pyramidal and other neural elements [78]. What is not clear is the range of fields that produce reversible neurological effects and the possible magnitude of induced changes. Our laboratory is currently investigating the effects of a variety of photo-magnetic, and microenergy wave forms on nerve conduction. Early progress is extremely encouraging, and we now believe that anesthesiology in the forthcoming century will undoubtedly offer the possibility of analgesia and regional anesthesia as well as sedation, hypnosis, and complete general anesthesia without a foreign compound via computer-focused physical activation of receptor sites and/or neurotransmitter modulation with noninvasive external wave forms or energy sources.

REFERENCES

1. Yaksh TL, Rudy TA. 1976. Analgesia mediated by direct spinal action of narcotics. Science 192:1357–1358.
2. Yaksh TL, Rudy TA. 1977. Studies on the direct spinal action of narcotics in the production of analgesia in the rat. J Pharmacol Exp Ther 202:411–428.
3. Wang JK, Nauss LA, Thomas JE. 1979. Pain relief by intrathecally applied morphine in man. Anesthesiology 59:149–151.
4. Kitahata LM, Collins JG. 1981. Spinal action of narcotic analgesics. Anesthesiology 54: 153–163.
5. Yaksh TL. 1981. Spinal opioid analgesia: Characteristics and principles of action. Pain 11: 293–346.
6. Cousins MJ, Mather LE. 1984. Intrathecal and epidural administration of opioids. Anesthesiology 61:276–310.
7. Yaksh TL, Hammond DL. 1982. Peripheral and central substances involved in the rostrad transmission of nociceptive information. Pain 13:1–86.
8. Cousins MJ, Mather LE, Glynn CJ, Wilson PR, Graham JR. 1979. Selective spinal analgesia. Lancet i:1141–1142.
9. Chauvin M, Samaii K, Schermann JM, et al. 1981. Plasma pharmacokinetics of morphine after intramuscular, extradural and intrathecal administration. Br J Anaesth 54:843–847.

10. Nordberg G, Hedner T, Mellstrand T, Dahlström B. 1984. Pharmacokinetics of epidural morphine in man. Eur J Clin Pharm 26:233–237.
11. Gourlay GK, Cherry DA, Cousins MJ. 1985. Cephalad migration of morphine in CSF following lumbar epidural administration in patients with cancer pain. Pain 23:317–326.
12. Nordberg G, Hedner T, Mellstrand T, Dahlström B. 1983. Pharmacokinetic aspects of epidural morphine analgesia. Anesthesiology 58:545–551.
13. Fromme GA, Steidl LF, Danielson DR. 1985. Comparison of lumbar and thoracic epidural morphine for relief of postthoracotomy pain. Anesth Analg 64:454–455.
14. Shulman M, Sandler A, Bradley JW, et al. 1984. Postthoracotomy pain and pulmonary function following epidural and systemic morphine. Anesthesiology 61:569–575.
15. Horan CT, Beeby DG, Brodsky JB, Oberhelman HA. 1985. Segmental effect of lumbar epidural hydromorphone: A case report. Anesthesiology 62:84–85.
16. Oden RV, Millar WL, Reisner LS. 1985. Epidural space pressures during continuous epidural fentanyl infusion. Anesthesiology 63 (Suppl): A252.
17. Lanz E, Kehrberger E, Theiss D. 1985. Epidural morphine: A clinical double-blind study of dosage. Anesth Analg 64:786–791.
18. Allen PD, Walman T, Concepcion M, et al. 1986. Epidural morphine provides postoperative pain relief in peripheral vascular and orthopedic surgical patients. A dose-response study. Anesth Analg 65:165–170.
19. Parker EO, Brookshire GL, Bartel SJ, et al. 1985. Effects of epinephrine on epidural fentanyl, sufentanil and hydromorphone for postoperative analgesia. Anesthesiology 63 (Suppl):A235.
20. Rawal N, Wattwil M. 1984. Respiratory depression after epidural morphine — an experimental and clinical study. Anesth Analg 63:8–14.
21. Lomessy A, Magnin C, Viale J-P, et al. 1984. Clinical advantage of fentanyl given epidurally for postoperative analgesia. Anesthesiology 61:466–469.
22. Oyama T. 1984. Effects of intrathecal and epidural morphine on endocrine function. In Estafanous FG (ed): Opioids in Anesthesia. Boston: Butterworth, pp. 75–79.
23. Lin DM, Shapiro HM, Shipko EM. 1985. Comparison of epidural lidocaine and fentanyl on spinal cord metabolism during sensory stimulation. Anesthesiology 62 (Suppl):A232.
24. Poletti CE, Cohen AM, Todd DP, Ojemann RG, Sweet WH, Zervas NT. 1981. Cancer pain relieved by long-term epidural morphine with permanent indwelling systems for self-administration. J Neurosurgy 55:581–584.
25. Chrusbasik J, Wiemers K. 1985. Continuous-plus-on-demand epidural infusion of morphine for postoperative pain relief by means of a small, externally worn infusion device. Anesthesiology 62:263–267.
26. Raj P, Knarr D, Vigdorth E, et al. 1985. Comparative study of continuous epidural infusions versus systemic analgesics for postoperative pain relief. Anesthesiology 63 (Suppl):A238.
27. Gustafsson LL, Post C, Edvardsen, Ramsay CH. 1985. Distribution of morphine and meperidine after intrathecal administration in rat and mouse. Anesthesiology 63:483–489.
28. Payne R, Inturrisi CE. 1985. CSF distribution of morphine, methadone and sucrose after intrathecal injection. Life Sci 37:1137–1144.
29. Bullingham RES, McQuay JH, Moore RA. 1982. Recent Advances in Anesthesia and Analgesia Edinburgh: Churchill Livingstone.
30. Glass PSA, Biagi B, Sischy S, Camporesi E. 1985. Analgesic action of very low dose intrathecal morphine (0.1 mg) as compared to higher doses (0.2–9.4 mg). Anesthesiology 63 (Suppl):A236.
31. Dailey PA, Brookshire GL, Schnider SM, et al. 1985. The effects of naloxone associated with the intrathecal use of morphine in labor. Anesth Analg 64:658–666.
32. Coombs DW, Fratkin JD, Meier FA, et al. 1985. Neuropathologic lesions and CSF morphine concentrations during chronic continuous intraspinal morphine infusion. A clinical and postmortem study. Pain 22:337–351.
33. Gibaldi M, Kanny JL. 1965. Drug absorption and the oral mucosa. J Oral Ther Pharmacol 1:440–445.
34. Watson J, Moore A, McQuay H, et al. 1984. Plasma morphine concentrations and analgesic effects of lumbar extradural morphine and heroin. Anesth Analg 63:629–634.
35. Paterson GMC, McQuay JH, Bullingham RES, Moore RA. 1984. Intradural morphine and diamorphine: Dose–response studies. Anaesthesia 39:113–117.
36. Merskey H. 1983. Diamorphine (heroin) and cancer pain. Can Med Assoc J 129:931–932.

37. Sawe J, Hansen J, Ginman G, et al. 1981. Patient controlled dose regimen for methadone for chronic cancer pain. Br Med J 282:771–773.
38. Evron S, Samueloff A, Simon A, et al. 1985. Urinary function during epidural analgesia with methadone and morphine in post-Cesarean section patients. Pain 23:135–144.
39. Yaksh TL, Noueihed R, Durant PA. 1984. Preliminary studies on the antinociceptive effects of intrathecal alfentanil in animal models. In Estafanous FG (ed): Opioids in Anesthesia. Boston: Butterworth, pp. 161–166.
40. Wen HL, Mehal ZD, Ong BH, et al. 1985. Intrathecal administration of beta-endorphin and dynorphine-(1–13) for the treatment of intractable pain. Life Sci 37:1213–1220.
41. Murphy DF. 1985. Epidural buprenorphine for postoperative pain relief (letter). Anesth Analg 64:456–463.
42. Lanz E, Simko G, Theiss D, Glocke M. 1984. Epidural buprenorphine — a double blind study of postoperative analgesia and side effects. Anesth Analg 63:593–598.
43. DeCastro J, Lecron L. 1981. Peridurale opiat-analgesie. Verschiedene opiate. Kimplikationen und nebenwirkungen. In Zenz M (ed): Peridurale opiat-analgesie. Stuttgart–New York: Fischer, pp.103–128.
44. Castillo RA, Kissin I, Bradley EL, 1986. Opioid agonist for spinal analgesia without risk of respiratory depression. Anesth Analg 65 (Suppl):S28.
45. Ling GSF, Spiegel K, Nishimura SL, Pasternak GW. 1983. Dissociation of morphine's analgesic and respiratory depressant action. Eur J Pharmacol 86:487–488.
46. Kalia PK, Madan R, Saksena R, et al. 1983. Epidural pentazocine for postoperative pain relief. Anesth Analg 62:949–950.
47. Weintraub SJ, Naulty JS. 1985. Acute abstinence syndrome after epidural injection of butorphanol. Anesth Analg 64:452–453.
48. Smith DJ, Perotti JM, Mansell AL, Monroe PJ, 1985. Ketamine analgesia is not related to an opiate action in the periaqueductal gray region of the rat brain. Pain 21: 253–265.
49. Finck AD, Ngai SH. 1982. Opiate receptor mediation of ketamine analgesia. Anesthesiology 56:291–297.
50. Bion JF. 1984. Intrathecal ketamine for war surgery. A preliminary study under field conditions. Anaesthesia 39:1023–1028.
51. Islas J, Astorga J, Laredo M. 1985. Epidural ketamine for control of postoperative pain. Anesth Analg 64:1161–1162.
52. Franz DN, Hare BD, McCloskey KL. 1982. Spinal sympathetic neurones: Possible sites of opiate withdrawal suppression by clonidine. Science 215:1643–1645.
53. Milne B, Cervenko FW, Jhamandas K, Sutak M. 1985. Intrathecal clonidine: Analgesia and effect on opiate withdrawal in the rat. Anesthesiology 62:34–38.
54. Taiwo YO, Fabian A, Pazoles CJ, Fields HL. 1985. Potentiation of morphine antinociception by monoamine re-uptake inhibitors in the rat spinal cord. Pain 21:239–337.
55. Milne B, Cervenko F, Jhamandas K, et al. 1985. Analgesia and tolerance to intrathecal morphine and norepinephrine infusion via implanted mini-osmotic pumps in the rat. Pain 22:165–172.
56. Coombs, DW, Saunders RL. Lachance D, et al. 1985. Intrathecal morphine tolerance: Use of intrathecal clonidine, DADLE, and intraventricular morphine. Anesthesiology 62:358–363.
57. Whitman JG. 1983. Benzodiazepine receptors. Anaesthesia 38:93–95.
58. Yaksh TL. 1982. Central and peripheral mechanisms for the antianalgesic action of acetylsalicyclic acid. In Barnett HJM, Hirsh J, Mustard JF (eds): Acetylsalicyclic Acid: New Uses for an Old Drug. New York: Raven Press, pp. 137–151.
59. Hokfelt T, Skirboll L, Lundberg JM, et al. 1983. Neuropeptides and pain pathways. In Bonica JJ (ed): Advances in Pain Research and Therapy. New York: Raven Press, pp. 227–246.
60. Chrubasik J, Meynadier J, Blond S, et al. 1984. Somatostatin, a potent analgesic. Lancet 8413:1208–1209.
61. Chrubasik J, Meynadier J, Scherpereel P. 1985. Somatostatin versus morphine in epidural treatment after major abdominal operations. Anesthesiology 63 (Suppl):A237.
62. Meynadier J, Chrubasik J, et al. 1985 Intrathecal somatostatin in terminally ill patients. A report of two cases. Pain 23:9–12.
63. Chrubasik J, Meynadier J, Scherpereel P, Wunsch E. 1985. The effect of epidural somatostatin on postoperative pain. Anesth Analg 64:1085–1088.
64. Baver W, Brainer U, Dopner W, et al. 1982. SMS 201–995: A very potent and selective

octapeptide analogue of somatostatin with problonged action. Life Sci 31:1133–1141.
65. Lamberts SWJ, Vitterlinden P, Verschoor L. 1985. Long-term treatment of acromegaly with the somatostatin analogue SMS-995. N Engl J Med 313:1576–1580.
66. Stanley TH, Leysen JE, Niemegeers CJ, Pace NL. 1983 Narcotic dosage and central nervous system opiate receptor binding. Anesth Analg 62:705–709.
67. Bangham AD. 1981. Introduction. Chapter 1. In Knight (ed): Liposomes: From Physical Structure to Therapeutic Applications. The Hague: Elsevier/North-Holland Biomedical Press.
68. Bangham AD. 1983. Liposomes in mice. Biol Cell 47:1–10.
69. Kirkpatrick A, Johansson J, Fiserova-Bergerova Y. 1985. Ultra-long local anesthesia with lecithin-coated methoxyflurane. Anesthesiology 63:A218.
70. Pasternak GW, Childers SR, Snyder SH. 1980. Naloxazone, a long-acting opiate antagonist: Effects of analgesia in intact animals and opiate receptor in binding in vitro. J Pharmacol Exp Ther 214:455–462.
71. Wofsy D. 1985. Strategy for treating autoimmune disease with monoclonal antibodies. West J Med 143:804–809.
72. Limoge A, Cara A, Debras C. 1978. Electrotherapeutic Sleep and Electroanesthesia. Paris: Masson.
73. Leduc S. 1903. L'electrisation cerebrale. Arch Elec Med 11:403–410.
74. Sjolund B, Ericksson M. 1976. Electro-acupuncture and endogenous morphines. Lancet ii:1085.
75. Stanley TH, Cazaloa JA, Atinault A, Cozytaux R, Limoge A, Louville Y. 1962. Transcutaneous cranial electrical stimulation decreases narcotic requirements during neuroleptanesthesia and operation in man. Anesth Analg 61:863–866.
76. Standley TH, Cazaloa JA, Limoge A, Louville Y. 1982. Transcutaneous cranial electrical stimulation increases the potency of N_2O in man. Anesthesiology 57:293–297.
77. Vander Ark GD, McGrath KA. 1975. Transcutaneous electrical stimulation in treatment of postoperative pain. Am J Surg 130:338–340.
78. Hause L, Sances A, Larson S. 1971. Polarization changes induced in the pyramidal cell and other neural elements by externally applied fields. In Wielfsohn NL, Sances A (eds): The Nervous System and Electrical Currents. New York: Plenum Press, pp. 93–95.

INDEX

Adverse effects of
  epidural opioids, 40, 50, 53
  intrathecal opioids, 40, 50
Affinity
  receptor, 2, 15, 21, 34, 36
Alfentanil, 20, 33, 135
Ambulation
  postoperative and epidural morphine, 46
Analgesia
  opioid receptors and, 20, 76
  patient controlled (PCA), 44
Analgesics
  adrenergic agents as, 54, 137
  agonist, 20, 34
  agonist/antagonist, 21
  antagonist, 22
  partial agonist, 22, 34
Antinociception
  animal studies, 34
Autoradiographic method
  receptor mapping for, 19

Baclofen
  epidural administration and spasticity, 44
Buprenorphine
  epidural, 21–23, 33, 136
Butorphanol
  epidural, 22

Caeserean section
  intraspinal opioids and, 105–108
  pain after, 104–109
Calcitonin
  epidural, 54
Cerebrospinal fluid (CSF)
  concentration of intraspinal opioids in, 37–38
  epidural drug transfer and, 37, 39
  intrathecal morphine and, 37–39
Chlornaltrexamine (β)
  epidural, 17
Chronic spinal analgesia
  drug delivery system, 115–127
  implanted ports, 119–122
  spinal catheter implantation, 116–119, 122–127
Clonidine
  intraspinal, 54, 137
Codeine, 22

DAGO, 14
Delta (δ) receptor, 16
Diamorphine
  epidural, 33
Drug transfer
  CSF and, 37
  vascular system and, 37
Dynorphin, 6–7, 11–12, 17–18

Endogenous opioids
  central distribution and, 9
Endorphin β, 6, 14, 79
Enkephalin, 6, 10, 14, 16
Epidural
  choice of non-opioids, 54
  choice of opioids, 43, 48–54, 130–132
  fat, 36
  intrathecal versus, 48–51, 130–132
  local anesthetic, 46
  local anesthetics and opioids, 56

Fentanyl
  epidural, 20, 22, 35, 51
Funaltrexamine (β), 14

Heroin
  intraspinal, 22, 135
Histopathological changes
  intraspinal opioids and, 52–54
Hydromorphone
  epidural, 33
Hydrophilic drugs
  intraspinal administration, 34, 53

Intercostal block
  epidural opioids and, 46
Intrapleural block, 45
Intraspinal opioids
  cost-benefit aspects, 46, 73–74
  ICU patients and, 48
  stress reduction and, 63–76
  see Epidural opioids
  see also Intrathecal opioids
Intrathecal opioids, 48–51, 133–134
  choice of drug, 51–54
Intravenous opioids, 36
Intraventricular drug administration, 36

Kappa (K) receptor, 17
Ketamine
  epidural, 54, 137
Ketocyclazocine, 17

Labor pain
  epidural opioids and local anesthetics
    and, 100–103
  epidural opioids in, 99–100
  intrathecal opioids and, 93–98

Levorphanol, 22
Lipophilic opioids
  respiratory depression and, 34, 51
Lofentanil
  epidural, 20, 22, 33–34, 36

Meperidine
  intraspinal administration, 22, 33, 36,
    51
Meptazinal
  epidural, 22
Methadone, 20, 22, 33, 52, 135
Midazolam
  epidural, 44, 54
Morphiceptin, 14
Morphine
  intramuscular, 45
  intraspinal, 20, 22, 33, 45, 51, 53
  intravenous, 45
Mu (μ) receptor, 14–16

Nalbuphine
  epidural, 22
Nalorphine, 22
Naloxonazine, 14
Naloxone, 14, 22
  reversal of adverse effects of
    intraspinal opioids and, 80–82
Neonatal effects
  intraspinal opioids and, 109–110
Neurotoxicity
  intraspinal opioids and, *see*
    Histopathology
Nociception
  Gate control theory and, 12
  opioid pathways and, 11
  spinal modulation and, 12

Obese patients
  analgesia and, 45
Obstetric analgesia
  intraspinal opioids and, 89–114
Opiates, *see* Opioids
Opioids
  aerosol, 44
  endogenous, 2
  epidural, *see* Epidural opioids
  exogenous, 2, 9
  intrathecal, *see* Intrathecal opioids
  oral controlled release, 44

pain pathways and, 11
patient controlled analgesia (PCA) and, 44
peptides and, 2, 7–9
pharmacology of, 21
sublingual, 44
transdermal, 44
transmucosal, 44
Oxymorphone
epidural, 22

Pain
cancer, 43
chronic, 43
herpes zoster, 43
myocardial infarction, 43
nephrolithiasis, 43
obstetric, 43, 89–114
perioperative, 43
postoperative, 33, 44
thrombophlebitis, 43
Partial agonists, 21, 23, 136
Patient controlled analgesia (PCA), 44–45
Peak expiratory flow
epidural morphine and, 46
Perioperative stress
intraspinal opioids and, 67–69
Pethidine, *see* Meperidine
Pharmacokinetics
intraspinal opioids and, 36–37
Phencycladine, 18
Placental transfer
epidural opioids and, 92
systemic opioids and, 91
Plasma concentration
epidural opioids and, 37
intrathecal opioids and, 37
Postoperative pain
intraspinal opioids, 20, 33
Pruritus
intraspinal opioids and, 78–79

Receptors
affinities and, 2, 15, 21, 34
binding sites of, 2
central distribution of, 19
classification of, 13–19

Sigma (σ) receptor, 18
Somatostatin
epidural, 54, 138
Spinal cord
distribution of opioid in, 39
histopathology and, 52–53
opioid distribution and, 39
spasticity and, 44
Stress
adrenocortical suppression and, 68
catecholamine release and, 68
endocrine/metabolic response and, 67–69
perioperative, 67–69
postoperative, 68, 70
reduction of, 66

Transdermal opioids, 44
Transmucosal opioids, 44
Traumatic pain
intraspinal opioids and, 46

Urinary retention
intraspinal opioids and, 79–82

Ventilatory depression, *see also* Respiratory depression
intraspinal opioids and, 40, 82–86

GPSR Compliance

The European Union's (EU) General Product Safety Regulation (GPSR) is a set of rules that requires consumer products to be safe and our obligations to ensure this.

If you have any concerns about our products, you can contact us on ProductSafety@springernature.com

In case Publisher is established outside the EU, the EU authorized representative is:

Springer Nature Customer Service Center GmbH
Europaplatz 3
69115 Heidelberg, Germany

Batch number: 10755292

Printed by Printforce, the Netherlands